GARY R. BICKFORD, PhD, FNP-BC
FAMILY NURSE PRACTITIONER

Our Stress is Killing Us:
*Money-back **Guaranteed** Solutions*

HEALTHY LIFE CLINIC, INC. ™

The opinions expressed in this manuscript are solely the opinions of the author and do not represent the opinions or thoughts of the publisher. The author has represented and warranted full ownership and/or legal right to publish all the materials in this book.

Our Stress is Killing Us: Money-back Guaranteed Solutions
All Rights Reserved.
Copyright © 2013 Gary R. Bickford, PhD, FNP-BC
v3.0 r.10

Cover Photo © 2013 JupiterImages Corporation.
All rights reserved - used with permission.

This book may not be reproduced, transmitted, or stored in whole or in part by any means, including graphic, electronic, or mechanical without the express written consent of the publisher except in the case of brief quotations embodied in critical articles and reviews.

Healthy Life Clinic, Inc. ™

ISBN: 978-0-578-12210-6

Library of Congress Control Number: 2013901508

PRINTED IN THE UNITED STATES OF AMERICA

Money-Back Guarantee If Not Satisfied!

(It takes twenty-one days to form a habit. If after thirty days of implementing the changes outlined in this book you are not better able to deal with undue stress, return the book with receipt and provide me contact information so I can discuss why this book did not help, and I will return your full purchase price.)

Table of Contents

Are We Stressed?	1
Do More	2
With Less	3
Faster	4
Spend Less Money	5
Increase Quality	7
Job Insecurity	8
Stress Awareness	9
Awareness of Stress in Ourselves	10
Our Body Will Lie to Us	14
Trigger to Recognize Undue Stress	17
Signs of Stress	19
Muscle Tension Increases	20
Digestion Slows	22
Sexual Interest Lowers	23
Breathing Rate Increases	27
Holmes-Rahe Stress Scale	29
Anxiety/Post Traumatic Stress Disorder (PTSD)	34
Irritability	35
Mental Fatigue	36
Avoiding Things	37
Going to Extremes	38
Administrative Problems	39
Legal Problems	40
Physical Signs	41

Illnesses	42
Physical Exhaustion	43
Reliance on Drugs	44
Ailments	45
Stomach Upset (milk allergy)	49
Chest Pain (go to ER)	50
Social Withdrawal (easier now with electronics)	51
Strategies	52
Physical Exam	53
Build Support Systems	55
Men Are Not As Good At This As Women	56
Choose Relationships to Build	58
Spend Time (Investment Time)	60
Quantity Time vs. Quality Time	61
Like You Just Saw the Person Yesterday Even After a Long Separation	62
Balance Activities	64
Work Should Not Be #1—If It Is Then You Have a Problem	66
Play	74
God and Family	76
Hobby	79
How to Balance - Increase Energy	81
Increase Success	83
What's Really Important?	96
What Happens/Worst Case?	98
Just Say NO!	101
Increase Energy	103
Exercise	105

2 to 1 payback	107
Push your body	109
Nutrition/Diet	110
Water	115
Reduce	127
Alcohol	128
Nicotine (Smoking Is Sooooooooo Stupid!)	132
Capillary Refill	137
Clubbing	139
YouTube Demo	140
Smoker's Cough	141
Caffeine	143
Sugar	147
Additives/Preservatives	149
Fruit for Breakfast	150
Do You Need to Lose Weight?	152
Fat	156
Adequate Sleep	157
Sleep Hygiene	162
Reduce TV	165
Time Management to Reduce Stress—Leave Early	166
Dictation Technology	167
Cell Phone	169
Music—Classical Reduces Beta-Endorphins	171
Audio Books	172
Safety	173
Hire Backup for Computer	179
Comedy/Laughter—Increases Alpha-Endorphins	180

Joke Books	181
Limit Immediate Access to Yourself	
(You Are Not That Important)	183
Money	185
Increase Rewards to Yourself	187
Large Rewards	188
Small Rewards	189
Vacations	190
Spiritual	192
Contact Friends	193
Be "Real"	194
Take Naps or Refreshing Breaks	201
Music	205
Forgive	207
Holiday Stressors	235
High Expectations	237
Positive Attitude	238
Love Runs Downhill	239
Smile—Embodied Cognition (Fake It Till You Make It)	241
Overcoming Sorrow	242
Increase Success - You Are Already Successful	244
Be a Decision Maker	245
Encourage Others	247
Write Notes	248
Phone Calls	249
Give, Give, and Give	250

Summary-Stress Is Both Positive and Negative	255
Increase Energy	256
Positive Attitude Toward Life	257
Reach Out	258
Be Good to Yourself	259
Use Stress to GROW!	260

Introduction

Very soon after graduating as a Family Nurse Practitioner (FNP-BC), I recognized that so many of the medical issues I was dealing with on a daily basis were caused by stress, and I enrolled in Vanderbilt University to gain further knowledge of how to deal with this major problem. That was a wonderful learning experience and has been very beneficial to me. I have continued to see patients and have had the opportunity to better serve them in helping them have healthier lifestyles and therefore contribute to a more satisfying, longer life.

I have studied and lectured on the impact of stress on our health for over twenty-six years. After giving the seminar under the title "Redirecting Stress" for about ten years for the DuPont Company, I copyrighted it under the same title in 1996, then continued to present it an additional sixteen years after copyright. I have been researching the subject for this book/seminar for all of this time, which would amount to over a quarter of a century. After retiring from over twenty years with the DuPont Company in medical diagnostics, I returned to graduate school to become a family nurse practitioner so I could serve the medically underserved.

I learned a great deal from the participants of the seminars that I presented in nearly every state in the U.S. The seminars were interactive and allowed the participants to comment during the seminar. Interestingly, the smaller audiences were the most interactive with the best sharing of experience in dealing with stress. The comments and questions from participants made the topic very "alive" to me and caused me to study even more about this important subject. My medical training and work experience as a family nurse practitioner really brought this subject home to me personally and allowed me to share with others the results of my long-term research. This long-term (approximately twenty-seven to thirty years) of study on how to deal with stress gives me the confidence in the suggestions enough to guarantee the results if the reader will put them into practice. I have seen many instances where so many of my patients have used these suggestions with excellent results. Just this week as I was entering a building to discuss opening a free medical clinic in the underserved area of Knoxville, Tennessee, a patient stopped me to tell me how his life had changed for the better due to some of these suggestions. It is so very humbling to know that suggestions I was able to make as a provider to the underserved were beneficial to this person's life. His expressions of gratitude were the highlight of my day!

Our stress *is* killing us (and others). It is increasing our blood pressure, causing insomnia, contributing greatly to anxiety and depression, causing us to eat improperly, to self-medicate with both legal and illegal drugs, driving us to financial ruin, and basically destroying our lives. Often we are not aware of the impact on our health and, therefore, our lives until we fully realize how we are improperly dealing with stress. Once we fully comprehend that stress is "very real" and is causing havoc in our lives, it is difficult to determine what we can do to minimize the impact of stress in our lives so we can truly enjoy ourselves.

Stress is actually good for us... It's when it is uncontrolled and not dealt with appropriately that we begin to have a problem. The only people who are not dealing with stress are dead! Everyone else has to deal with it not only daily but all day, every day.

The positive aspect to stress is that it causes us to perform as we should. The stress of being an adult and taking on an adult role

INTRODUCTION

in life motivates us in a very positive way to provide for our own needs, and if we have a family, then the stress of providing for them causes us to get moving to do what we need to do to provide all that we can for them.

The stress of a test in school makes us study better; the stress of having to deal with another speeding ticket helps us keep within the posted limits, at least most of the time. The stress of limited resources causes us to account for how we are spending/investing our money (even very wealthy people have limited resources).

So, if you are stressed, that is good, if it drives you to perform in an optimal fashion so you can have a fulfilled life that brings great satisfaction. The problem is when our stress is too great and is not dealt with adequately. This undue stress is damaging our health, emotions, and personal relationships and can negatively impact our careers.

This negative stress is best thought of as "distress." This negative stress is like having a ball and chain around both ankles. It certainly pulls us down as we are struggling so greatly to "survive" that we cannot enjoy our lives, and we are damaging our health.

There is even a term for too much positive stress! The term is "eustress," which is a combination of the words "euphoria" and "stress." There have been attempts to determine which of the two types of stress impact the body negatively the most. It appears that the impact on the body and everyday lives of the individual is approximately equal!

How could eustress be stressful? Good news can also cause undue stress to a level of negativism, *i.e.*, a new promotion or even a new job. If you receive that long-awaited promotion, there is great cause for celebration, but you and your family may be the only ones celebrating. More than likely your work peers will not be as thrilled for you as you might hope, so that is a stressor. Moving to the new position, which is a "growth" position for you, means you are now out of your comfort zone, plus you have many of your peers watching to see if you succeed or not. Often some of your peers will attempt to sabotage your success, especially if they are now reporting to you. So, your check may be bigger, but you will earn every penny of that increase.

Post Traumatic Stress Disorder (PTSD) is very real and is much more prevalent than most realize. This work reveals many ideas that will help **anyone** that is suffering from PTSD.

Are We Stressed?

It really is not a question of *if* we are stressed but *how much* we are stressed and even more important is how we are dealing with this stress. Where is the "threshold" of stress for each of us? Is mine lower or higher than yours? This is as difficult of a question as "Is my pain tolerance the same as yours?" We must realize where our critical point is, which stress is good for us to help us strive to better ourselves, and where it becomes toxic to our lives and keeps us from fulfilling our daily requirements of our work, family, and overall lifestyle. So, yes, we are all stressed, and most of the time that is beneficial, but once we cross our threshold, we must make some changes or we will become almost paralyzed in our ability to succeed.

Do More

In our society of faster and faster communication, we are expected to do more than ever before. Each effort or "production run" is to be done with more productive work. One of the disadvantages of so much information about the rest of the world is that we most often hear of the exceptions and compare our work with them rather than the information that may be more correct of the production results.

With Less

Not only are we expected to do more, but we are expected to accomplish greater productivity while using fewer resources! It is much simpler to increase productivity if given adequate resources (money, personnel, and products), but today our society expects more from less. This is a very compounding problem, so if you are expected to produce 10% more with 10% fewer resources, then you now have a 20% difference between your productivity and resources. Since we often work five days a week, a 20% difference in our productive capabilities is like one extra day of work a week that we don't get paid for, and this extra work also encroaches on our "downtime" to deal with undue stress.

Faster

We have become so accustomed to instant communication and information that we are programmed to expect results as fast as we can communicate the results. We don't always realize that it took a great deal of time prior to the "announcement" in the media. Some writers say that we became programmed to crimes being solved in one hour or less due to watching the one-hour TV crime shows. In actuality, when you read of how long it takes to collect enough information to arrest someone, process them with the current system, and then actually deliver the final punishment, you begin to wonder if we will ever win against the criminals. It takes so many of our law enforcement officers and judicial system resources to gain a conviction on a crime that was spontaneous and only took a few minutes to commit.

We want results immediately in some areas of our life where it is impossible to achieve immediate results. Our lives are too complicated to make immediate changes without causing other parts of our life some stress. It takes three to four weeks to form a new habit, and it seems to take even longer to break a bad habit. Sometimes we do something positive in our lives to reduce our undue stress, but we still retain old habits that somewhat reduce the benefit of the new habit.

Spend Less Money

Our economy is affecting everyone, not only in the United States but worldwide. If you have more money to spend right now than you have had in the last several years, then you are very fortunate, because most people do not. Even the wealthy are struggling with the current economy, but we don't hear of that often or even think of that often because we feel that wealth insulates you from economic stress. If a middle-income person takes a 15% reduction in net worth, it could amount to from a few thousand to a few hundred thousand dollars, but to a person blessed with wealth; it could mean several million dollars. We have difficulty understanding how much the wealthy are impacted because we may not have that much money, and we may also not understand how much others are impacted who have less money than we do.

In my practice I have many patients who are on disability or unemployment or even social security, and their check is significantly less than a thousand dollars a month. On this amount of money they are to pay for rent, utilities, food, clothing, transportation, communication...etc. Most of my patients do not even have access to the Internet and do not know how to use it at free sites like the local library. Their cell phone is one where they just buy what minutes they can afford. Whenever we needed to call our patients about some change we needed to inform them of, usually less than a third had a working phone number or a way to leave a message.

We so often forget how much we have already because we compare ourselves with the "rich and famous." This is a problem with our society in that we hold those who have money or fame up too high and compare ourselves with them and feel that we are failures. That is unfair to ourselves. We need to recognize that we are already successful. If you have obtained a copy of this book, then you are successful enough to know about it and have the resources to obtain it by whatever means necessary.

Increase Quality

I remember years ago, when I would get a new company car while working for DuPont, I would put a notebook and pen in the car just to write down the problems so I would not miss anything when I took it back to the dealer one to two times just getting the manufacturing problems resolved. There was always something that the dealer needed to repair. Now when we get a new car (or any product), good quality is a given. "Made in Japan" was a part of many jokes during my earlier years until "made in Japan" came to mean high quality or well made. In our workforce today we are expected to deliver high quality in everything we do because our society does not accept less.

Job Insecurity

Job insecurity is a tremendous source of undue stress, and that level of insecurity is higher now than at any time in history. No one has a secure job today. Even if you win the lottery or inherit a great deal, your future is still not guaranteed. Our news services are full of stories of people who have made or received a great deal of money but for whatever circumstances no longer have that level of lifestyle. Even famous homes like the Vanderbilt's' Biltmore Estate and the Hearst Castle can only exist as museums because the maintenance costs are too great to keep them as viable homes.

For a male, being out of a job is one of the greatest stressors we experience! One of the first questions men ask each other is "What kind of work do you do?" To say that we are unemployed or looking for work is very difficult, especially if we have had a good career thus far. It may not be fair that our work "defines" most men, but that is how many men feel.

If a woman is in a relationship where her partner is working and she loses her job, the stress is not so great due to a second income for the household, but if she is single, the impact could equal the men's. If she is a single mother, the threat of losing her job is even more stressful. I have had so many female patients relate that they are required to lift heavy objects at work but that they don't dare complain for fear of losing their job. Unemployment is not enough to live on, especially if you have not made much money to start with.

Stress Awareness

Stress is a cumulative process. Often we do not even realize how our stress level has progressed beyond the "threshold" of being a positive impact on our lives to a level that is toxic to practically all aspects of our life. It does not appear that our society is making it any easier for us to deal with our stress. Just the single aspect of "instant access" to us or the expectation from society to have instant access to us is extremely stressful, and undermines much of our attempts to reduce our stress to a positive level. Others expect an immediate response from us, and we often catch ourselves expecting the same of others.

Awareness of Stress in Ourselves

Forgive me for relating too much personal information about myself, but I know the details of my health issues due to stress better than I would anyone else's even if they were very open and frank about their situation.

During the time that my marriage was in real trouble, my wife mentioned to me that I was scratching my head a great deal more than usual. I was unaware of this change (as we are often of our changes due to stress), but I began noticing that what she said was true. I had never had a problem with dandruff (skin flaking off the scalp due to dryness), and I would have easily been aware because as a DuPont employee I wore mostly dark blue suits, which would have made a problem with dandruff readily apparent.

I had excellent health insurance, so I called the dermatologist I had seen for years due to some minor skin damage from the multiple times I was badly sunburned as a child. I saw him often and had an annual skin "tune-up" to minimize any further damage to my fair complexion.

When I told him what my wife had said and that I had never had a dandruff problem, he began to examine my scalp by holding his hand level and starting at my neck, moving his hand upward to allow my hair to drop off his hand as he did so. This method of examining the scalp allows the provider to have a clear look at the skin below the hair. (I now use his technique when I examine my own patients with scalp complaints.)

He said that I had several dry areas on my scalp that had not begun to flake yet but would do so soon without treatment. He surprised me by asking what was going on in my life to cause me to be so stressed! I actually had to think what could be causing me to be stressed. I told him that I was really struggling with my marriage and it appeared that divorce was imminent. Also, I had been asked to present a seminar in Hawaii in a few months on a subject that was new to me, and I was concerned that I might not have time to prepare adequately.

This dermatologist further surprised me by telling me that he sees this same skin condition in accountants around tax filing time, teachers near the end of the school year, and law enforcement or military employees when they change to more dangerous assignments. So his advice was to just use over-the-counter (OTC) medications for dandruff if the flaking started, but in the meantime attempt to reduce or better handle my stress.

In addition to the skin manifestations of my stress level, I also began having difficulty breathing some of the time. I know that this is a common occurrence in panic attacks, but I didn't feel that I was having that problem. But something was causing a difficulty with breathing at times. So I went to see a pulmonologist for an evaluation. I have never smoked but was around secondhand smoke while growing up. Everything checked out fine with this specialist.

As I mentioned earlier I have given seminars for years for DuPont and really enjoyed meeting the many wonderful people while doing so. Now something really scary started happening to me. My voice started becoming hoarse, so the sound of it was changing even with normal conversation. There were two reasons why this health condition was such a concern, with the second one even greater than the first. My job was to sell (marketing is a more sophisticated term for selling that we often use when we are selling very expensive, high-end equipment), so my income could be jeopardized if I was not able to communicate appropriately with my prospects and seminar participants. I had two young daughters at this time as well as a wife, so I needed to keep my income where it was, at least. The second reason was much more of a concern. My father was diagnosed with throat cancer several years before and had undergone extensive radiation to kill the cancer cells. He was a heavy smoker and smoked in the house where we lived, so I had inhaled his secondhand smoke all of my early life. When the term "cancer" is used, everything becomes much more serious, and I can understand how devastating it is to hear that term used by your provider.

Much of the reason I chose to be a nurse practitioner (or midlevel) provider is because I never wanted to have to tell any patient that they had cancer just because of how that term changes their life forever. I remember so very well the first patient I referred to a specialist who I felt had cancer. I certainly did not tell her my suspicions because I feel strongly that this level of diagnosis should <u>only</u> be made by a MD and preferably one who specializes in that area of concern. When the specialist sent me his report on her, stating that she was already in stage IV (the worst stage), I was terrified about telling her of his report. I called the specialist (surgeon) to confirm the report was correct and to solicit his advice on how to approach this 20-year-old patient. Fortunately, he related that he had already informed her! What a stress relief that was to me. He already had her scheduled for surgery and chemotherapy. She has made a full recovery at the last report and continued to see me for some time afterward.

So now that I was experiencing the persistent hoarseness, I headed to an ear, nose, and throat (ENT) specialist. After a quick exam he said I had a polyp on one of my vocal cords and that was causing the change in my voice. He could not comment on whether it was cancerous until he removed the tissue and sent it to the pathologist for diagnosis. We scheduled the surgery almost immediately due to my concern about my father's throat cancer. The tissue that was removed was benign (non-cancerous), so I did not have to continue worrying about cancer. That was another wonderful relief, but in about three months after the surgery and a lack of hoarseness, the change in my voice came back. Cancer cells are very fast-growing cells, so again that concern had reared its ugly head. When I was reexamined I was told that the polyp was back.

Since it came back in such a short time, I lost confidence in that specialist and consulted with another ENT here in Knoxville. When he examined my throat, he said yes there was a polyp, but he did not want to do surgery again due to the fragility of the thin, muscular vocal cord. He referred me to a specialist at Vanderbilt Hospital who dealt with similar problems with the many singers who worked in the Nashville, Tennessee, area in the country western music business.

This Vanderbilt specialist also saw the polyp but felt it looked benign from his experience and the earlier pathology reports. Again, I was very surprised when he said, "What is going on in your life?" I told him that I was very concerned about throat cancer, my hoarseness negatively impacting my career, as well as an impending divorce. He said that at night just enough gastric fluid was refluxing up my esophagus to irritate my vocal cords but not enough to awaken me. His treatment was a medicine for acid reflux, and he suggested that I reduce the stress in my life or learn how to handle it better. I took the prescription medications for about three months as well as his other advice and have never had the problem again.

So here were several different manifestations in my life in how my undue stress was very negatively impacting my health. If you were to have asked me during this time if I was overly stressed, I would have told you that I did have some stress but I was handling it appropriately. Now, it is obvious that I was not handling my overload of stress nearly as well as I perceived that I was.

Our Body Will Lie to Us

Soon after realizing that I was not dealing with my stress well enough, I found out that we can't always trust our body or thoughts to tell us the truth about our true health situation. After my divorce, for several mornings I noticed a small amount of blood on the sheet near my upper back area. Since I was single I did not have anyone I could ask to examine my back to determine the source of the blood, so off I went to my dermatologist again.

He had me remove my shirt and while poking and prodding on my back, he said, "Now, Gary, don't worry about this. It is just a basal cell carcinoma. They are the safest of the carcinomas, and I will just cut this out and send it to pathology. Call me back on Monday (four days later) and I will give you the path results." There again when <u>anyone</u> hears carcinoma, they think cancer no matter how you attempt to sugar-coat the phrase.

However, since I had been doing so much better handling my stress from the earlier physical problems and all of them had abated, I felt that I could deal with this also. I knew that basal cell carcinoma was the safest of the skin cancers, and that usually when the tissue is removed, the problem is gone forever. The next step up the cancer line is squamous cell carcinoma, but even that is not as bad as melanoma, which is the most serious of the three levels of skin cancer. The dermatologist told me he had taken a good-sized sample and for me not to worry.

I left his office with confidence in what he had said, and I was convinced that I was not worried about cancer being a problem since my earlier problems were now gone. I knew that I had more than adequate life insurance and that I was worth a great deal more dead than alive, so I knew my children would be adequately provided for if something did happen to me. I also felt that my ex-wife would not have a difficult time dealing with my death unless she hurt herself when she was jumping for joy.

People who know me well might not think I am going to Heaven, but I have a faith that allows me to feel confident that while I am nowhere near perfect, I can feel secure in knowing that I am forgiven for my problems. So that part was not a problem for me. We often ask for prayers from other believers, and certainly cancer is a time you would want to consider that request, but I did not in this case because of my conviction that if this was basal cell carcinoma it had been removed and we were done with that.

I did tell my sister, who is more than just a sister—she is also one of my very closest friends on this earth. She has been an angel to me all of her life, and I don't understand why, because I used to torment her terribly when we were younger. She was my favorite target! The only thing I ever did for her as a youngster was to give her a blank check to go get a prom dress every year she went. She was always judicious in her spending and still looked wonderful for that special night each year.

So, on Monday after the tissue specimen was taken on Thursday, I called the dermatologist, who said, "I was incorrect about my initial diagnosis."

One thing you learn when you are a provider of healthcare to others is that you have to be extremely careful of everything you say to a patient when you are talking about a diagnosis of their health. Patients always assume the worst, and once they hear the negative, they don't hear the positive side of the problem. So, my first thought was that the path report was worse than the basal cell carcinoma. He quickly went on to say, "It was just a severely infected hair follicle." He instructed me to come to his office in three or four days to have the sutures removed where he had taken the specimen.

What was so very devastating to me and rocked me to my heels was how much my shoulders relaxed when I received this wonderful news! I could not believe it! It seemed that my shoulders dropped an inch, and I could take a full breath. I was absolutely humbled, and shocked, that I could be that stressed while convincing myself that I was not worried about this potential cancer scare. That was almost 20 years ago, but I can remember it like it was just yesterday—how I was able to fool myself into a certainty of "no worries" when my body externally was so very obviously super-stressed just by the immediate relaxation of my upper body and the deep breath I was able to take. Maybe you have had a similar experience(s), but that was my first that I deeply remember, and it definitely convinced me that I could not trust myself to correctly ascertain what my stress level truly is. I regret giving so much detail here, but if it helps a reader better understand their stress level, then I am willing to "open my kimono" to share anything that might be of benefit to others.

Trigger to Recognize Undue Stress

Everyone needs to determine what their "trigger" or physical change that makes you aware of how your stress level is beginning to cause problems. It can be anything that makes you aware. For some it is an eye tic; others report wringing of hands or tapping of pen on desk. For me, it is the trapezius muscle on the left side of my back. When it begins to tighten up enough that I am aware of the feeling, I know that my stress is getting to me. This helps me to start looking at ways to reduce my stress or to determine what is causing me more stress than usual. If it begins to "burn," I know I need to do something soon. If the left side is burning and then I can feel the same muscle on the right side of my back begin to tighten up enough that I can feel it, then I know I need to stop what I am doing, and do something quickly about my stress level.

When my trigger is telling me I am stressed, this is not always a bad thing. I have found that anytime I am speaking about any subject, my trigger is in full force, but that is understandable due to the natural stress of giving seminars. I have given at least two seminars where I felt no stress signals, and they were my two worst presentations from my standpoint as well as determined from the audience survey. The normal stress comes from wanting to do a good job for the audience so as not to waste their valuable time; the fear of saying something inappropriate accidently; the concern that something I may say innocently might offend someone else's sensitivities; the concern of going too long, being boring, jokes or humor falling flat, a crooked tie, not getting my points across, falling down as I move about, having an appropriate volume, not speaking too rapidly, sounding cosmopolitan (so people cannot determine what part of the country I am from which can detract from the message), ...etc

I absolutely love giving seminars because I have been speaking publically all of my adult life and several years as a teenager. The speaking just comes naturally to me and has from the very beginning, so I normally just have to be concerned about the content of the discussion. Still, I need to know that I am under pressure in order to perform the best I can for the audience. I never feel that I have done a good job because the audience deserves an outstanding speaker and interesting subject matter; they are honoring any speaker by taking time and making the effort to listen to them. I often have flown or driven for several hours to give a short talk, and I dislike the "wear and tear" on my body, but when I feel the audience has gained at least one thing that could benefit them, now or later, I forget the difficulties of the travel. So when I am giving a seminar, I want my trigger to let me know that I have stress and need to do a good job, but I don't want it to burn or move to the right side because my undue stress could detract from my efforts.

Signs of Stress

We need to be aware of signs of stress that indicate that we are not handling our undue stress appropriately in ourselves and in others. These signs can be useful if we are able to intervene in our own stress levels as well as those who are important to us. Helping others recognize and deal with their stress can even contribute to lowering our own stress level. If we know this other person well enough to observe their stress signs, then that person must be important to us.

The American Psychological Association's "Stress in America" report released in 2010 lists common effects on your body, mood, and behavior as follows: <u>Body</u>—headache, muscle tension or pain, chest pain, fatigue, change in sex drive, stomach upset, sleep problems; <u>Mood</u>—anxiety, restlessness, lack of motivation or focus, irritability or anger, sadness or depression; <u>Behavior</u>—overeating or undereating, angry outbursts, drug or alcohol abuse, tobacco abuse, and social withdrawal. Sometimes we feel that we are experiencing **all** of this list plus others that are not mentioned!

Muscle Tension Increases

Muscle tension is definitely a reaction to excessive stress. I see so many patients who are dealing with headaches due to or exacerbated by stress. One of the most defining questions to ask someone about their headaches is to ask what time of day they come on. If the answer is later in the day, then most often those are tension headaches caused by stress. The patients often describe the pain as beginning in their head and then progressing down to the back of the neck. Both of these pains can be caused by the tension of muscles or spasms.

Migraine headaches can come on any time of the day but are not usually consistent in their timing of later in the day. One can even have both types of headaches where both are impacted by the stress that manifests itself in the musculature of the body. Migraines can hit you at any time and can be completely debilitating. I suffered from migraines from my late teens to my mid-forties. It was extremely hard on my wife and children to have to deal with my not being able to attend some very important functions that we had planned for months. Many people have told me that they had severe migraines and they just went to a quiet place or maybe took two aspirin and they went away. I would tell them that they might have had a headache, but it probably was not a migraine because that usually does not work with a migraine. Migraines usually come with nausea or vomiting, photophobia (increased pain associated with light), and/or a greatly increased sense of hearing.

Fortunately, a medicine came along that was a miracle drug for me. At first it was only available as an injection, but it is now available as an injection, which works the fastest; nasal spray (the next fastest); and tablet form. The drug is Imitrex® and is now generic so it is easier to get your insurance to pay for it. If you are having migraine-type headaches and your provider has not allowed you to try this type of medicine, then find one who will. If it works for you, you will agree that it is at least an "almost miracle" drug. There are others in that family of drugs, but they all compare to Imitrex as a standard. That medicine gave me my life back! I had some in every car, office, and desk that I used as well as carried it in my pocket.

At one time before that medicine came along, I was averaging one day a week where I was not able to work. Most of that time I worked out of an office at home, so I was able to rearrange my schedule and sleep all day to recover from the strong drugs I had to take to overcome the pain and nausea. It is common for migraine sufferers to find that the frequency of the headaches greatly decrease or go completely away in the mid-forties to mid-fifties as mine have now. I used to always have to plan for the next day what I would do if I did not have a migraine and how I would attempt to keep my job if I had to sleep all day. If I had had a regular office job during all those years, I am confident I would have been fired for missing so much work. I am blessed that I was able to even keep a good job during that part of my life. With that experience of migraines for so many years, I am confident that stress contributed to them, but they were not caused by stress. I am more stressed now than ever in my life, and I have not had a migraine in years. Many migraines are familial (genetic based), as mine were; my maternal grandfather and my mother also had severe migraine headaches.

Digestion Slows

Stress can cause your digestion to take much longer processing the food you have consumed to be used for energy. There are some very important aspects to realize about digestion that impact your ability to deal with the stressors of life. One aspect is that it takes energy to digest the food you have just eaten; up to about ten percent of the caloric value of the food ingested is used in the digestion process. Plus it takes hours for the food to become energy. Food does not become energy until it is in the small intestine, where the millions of villi absorb the nutrients the digestion system has prepared in the stomach. Thus you can gain energy from food you consumed some time ago. This process takes longer than most of us realize, and if it is often further delayed due to stress, then it is like attempting to drive your car with no fuel in the tank. We will discuss this further later when we discuss how to overcome some of the stress. It can help you plan your eating times when you fully realize that it takes several hours to digest a full meal.

Sexual Interest Lowers

Now this is an important topic! Stress can certainly cause our interest to diminish in sex and/or any other pleasurable activity. Sex can be a wonderful stress reliever but only if you feel good about the activity and are not distracted by the undue stress in your life. When a mother has small children she is almost totally responsible for, this constant stress can cause her to lose interest in having any fun. This constant pressure to keep the children safe is enough stress just by itself, not even considering feeding, clothing, and bathing them. No matter how diligent you are as a parent, your children will get into potentially dangerous situations.

I had to perform the Heimlich maneuver on both of my daughters. My older daughter was two or three years old when she was playing while eating part of an apple. My younger daughter was only three months old. My younger daughter was born with teeth, and we were visiting with another couple who had a baby of similar age. They had been giving their daughter teething biscuits, which were safe because their baby did not have teeth. My daughter was able to bite off a good-sized chunk that blocked her airway. Once we realized she was in danger, I laid her over my fist, pounded on her back twice, and pushed her down further on my fist. She expelled the piece of biscuit easily and did not even become upset with the maneuver. Needless to say, the rest of us adults had to take a break to settle down. Most parents who have reared children to adulthood firmly believe in "angels watching over our children."

Mothers who stay at home with little to no adult conversation all day long begin to focus on the mother role more than their other role as a wife, and for good reason. The pressure on a mother is tremendous, and they only have a certain amount of energy. Sometimes the mother could benefit from telling their spouse, "Right now most of my energy has to be focused on the children, but if you will assist me in their care, I will have more energy to spend on **us**." The father who does not interact with his children is losing some of the most interesting and fun times of their lives as well as the memories that would bring enormous comfort later in life.

Fathers who are so stressed at work can also lose pleasure in activities that have brought great pleasure in the past. Certainly there are medical problems that can reduce interest in sexual activities, and these should be ruled out also. While it is recognized that it is very stressful to be a mother, it is also stressful to be a father. Sometimes that stress is positive because it can make fathers mature more after having a child than they might have in the past. The undue stress of having to provide for children and family can reduce our pleasure of life when we begin to feel overwhelmed.

Men also have the stress of "security" for their family to assure that they are not in danger from outsiders. I remember my older daughter looking around in a small restaurant owned by some of my best friends and then asking, "Why are all the men facing the front of the restaurant and all the women facing the back?" She seemed surprised when I told her that it was a "man thing" due to the responsibility of protecting their family. That is also why men usually sit to the outside on the aisle seats so they will be able to move quickly as well as have their family as far from any potential danger as possible that would probably come from the aisle area.

Men also have the burden of society expecting them to protect any woman or child even if they do not know them. If one man is in the company of several women and/or children when there is some sort of danger to the group, every male (father, husband, brother, son, grandson, grandfather) in each of the women's lives expect the man to do all that he can to protect them. All the men would want to know what the man did to protect them and would expect him to place himself in harm's way to minimize the danger, even to the point of physical damage to the male. Men expect other men to be prepared to defend the women and children to the point where it is physically impossible to resist any further and even be willing to give their life if necessary.

There have been numerous surveys of families who report they are happy after decades of marriage, and most of them report having a "date night" at least every two weeks as very important in keeping the relationship healthier. The date night includes finding someone to feed, babysit, and get the children to sleep so the parents can have several hours of uninterrupted time together. Often the date is just time away from home without the children and without it being an expensive dinner date.

I see many older patients who are now rearing grandchildren without the help of the parents of the children. Often the parents are just not ready to accept the responsibility of taking care of the children because the time interferes with their "party" lifestyle. The responsibility of rearing children should be on the young parents because as much as we grandparents love our grandchildren, we honestly don't have the energy to parent them appropriately.

Sometimes there is an aging parent in the home, which adds to the stress level and reduces interest in sexual activities. I also see many patients who are at the point of exhaustion due to the stress of attempting to be a full-time caregiver. It is called "caregiver strain" and most often the caregiver becomes ill due to the stress of keeping an older person 24/7. I often ask patients in this situation how many different shifts of people take care of patients in nursing homes. They respond with three full-time positions to take care of them plus at least one other full-time position to account for vacation and holidays. So a full-time caregiver is attempting to have the same diligence and focus as four full-time employees! I suggest that my patients put their elderly parents into a care facility and then they can go visit them every day and stay all day if they choose. So many patients have come back to see me with tears in their eyes, thanking me for the suggestion about care for the elderly person, because now the <u>patient</u> has their life back. Sometimes other siblings disagree with the patient's decision, so I suggest that they ask the ones who disagree with them when they want to take the elderly person into their home for continual care. Patients have also responded that this is also beneficial because now the complainers are much more understanding and agree with the decision.

So, if your spouse is not as interested in sexual activities, then you both may need to discuss your respective stress levels and how that might be affecting your lives. The suggestions found in this book could possibly increase your interest again in a very stress-relieving activity. Certainly the problem could be due to hormonal imbalances that can be verified with common laboratory testing. Even the levels can be impacted by undue stress, so the need for additional hormones may be temporary and might not show a consistent imbalance.

Breathing Rate Increases

One of the most useful methods to help a person who is anxious for any reason is to instruct them to breathe slower and deeper. It may even be helpful to ask them to breathe with you, to breathe deeply, involving abdominal muscles, and it may be instructive to place their hand along with yours on their abdomen to gauge the depth of the breathing. You may have to spend several minutes with the person working on their breathing to see the results and allow the patient to observe the difference.

One of my most humorous moments while working in the emergency department was doubly benefited from deep breathing. A nurse came to tell me that a patient was having a severe anxiety attack in the waiting room. When I arrived, the female patient was holding on to the back legs of one of the chairs while lying on the floor. She showed several signs of a panic attack, such as rapid breathing, trembling hands, dilated pupils, as well as rapid speech. So I kneeled down on the floor and asked her to start deep and slow breathing. That was very diagnostic, but also a mistake because her breath reeked of alcohol so much that I was in danger of testing positive for alcohol consumption myself! When I told her companions and the nursing staff that she was just drunk, they were so relieved. We admitted her to the ER, but she left before being seen by a provider. She really did not need to be taking up the ER time and space anyway. She was a GOMER (Get Out of My Emergency Room). She just needed time for the alcohol to be processed out of her body.

When we are stressed we also tend to take more shallow breaths, and this does not allow for adequate volume of air to flow. This flow of air allows the exchange of waste products in the lungs (carbon dioxide, CO_2) with the oxygen that the cells need to function appropriately. This oxygen is attached to the hemoglobin and circulates to the cells, where it is used as energy to keep the cells operating optimally. That is why anytime someone is in distress, you always check for proper ventilation (oxygenation) by confirming that their airway is open; then you need to make certain they are breathing adequately, and then you confirm that the heart is beating for circulation, because if there is not oxygen getting into the body, a beating heart will just be pushing blood that is of no use to the cells. This is the ABC of first-responders' code: Airway, Breathing, and Circulation.

Anytime you are feeling stressed, take a few seconds to assess your breathing. Are you breathing too fast and shallowly, thereby robbing your body of the oxygen it so desperately needs?

There are many chemical changes to the body during increased stress levels, and they are discussed by Joseph Shrand, MD from Harvard and his co-author, Leigh M. Devine, in their 2012 book entitled, *Manage Your Stress: Overcoming Stress in the Modern World*. What I am writing puts much more emphasis on *how* to deal with stress to stop or minimize these changes due to stress rather than the technical biological changes that these authors discuss so well.

Holmes-Rahe Stress Scale

In 1967, psychiatrists Thomas Holmes and Richard Rahe decided to study whether or not stress contributes to illness. They surveyed more than 5,000 medical patients and asked them whether they had experienced any of a series of forty-three life events in the previous two years. Each event, called a Life Change Unit (LCU), had a different "weight" for stress. The more events the patient added up, the higher the score. The higher the score, and the larger the weight of each event, the more likely the patient was to become ill.

Life Event	Life Change Units
Death of a spouse	100
Divorce	73
Marital separation	65
Imprisonment	63
Death of a close family member	63
Personal injury or illness	53
Marriage	50
Dismissal from work	47
Marital reconciliation	45
Retirement	45
Change in health of family member	44
Pregnancy	40
Sexual difficulties	39
Gain a new family member	39
Business readjustment	39

Change in financial state	38
Death of a close friend	37
Change to different line of work	36
Change in frequency of arguments	35
Major mortgage	32
Foreclosure of mortgage or loan	30
Change in responsibilities at work	29
Child leaving home	29
Trouble with in-laws	29
Outstanding personal achievement	28
Spouse starts or stops work	26
Begin or end school	26
Change in living conditions	25
Revision of personal habits	24
Trouble with boss	23
Change in working hours or conditions	20
Change in residence	20
Change in schools	20
Change in recreation	19
Change in church activities	19
Change in social activities	18
Minor mortgage or loan	17
Change in sleeping habits	16
Change in number of family reunions	15
Change in eating habits	15
Vacation	13
Christmas	12
Minor violation of law	11

Total score of 300+: At risk of illness in next two years

Score of 150-299: Risk of illness is moderate (reduced by 30% from the above risk)

Score <150: Slight risk of illness

Note: If you experienced the same event more than once, then to gain a more accurate total, add the score again for each extra occurrence of the event.

This table is taken from the Social Readjustment Rating Scale, Thomas H. Holmes and Richard H. Rahe, *Journal of Psychosomatic Research*, Volume 11, Issue 2, August 1967, Pages 213-218. The benefit of this being an older study (1967) is that it has been very well proven over the years to be accurate.

During my numerous lectures using this stress scale, I often related that I had not had a spouse die (100 points), but I had been through a divorce (73 points), and I felt these two numbers could justifiably be reversed. I had three participants at these different presentations tell me that they had experienced both the death of a spouse and a divorce, and they agreed that a divorce is more stressful than the death of a spouse. They all said the death has a "finality" to it, and you now tend to remember the better things about your former spouse, whereas a divorce is a continual, ongoing (almost always), unpleasant relationship that seldom improves with time. So the pain continues for years due to the broken relationship where both often focus on the negatives of their former spouse rather than remembering the more pleasant parts of that relationship.

I decided to take this stress test myself. That was not a good idea! My score was 262, not counting the stress of attempting to write this book! This book should have put me over the edge. My stress trigger was active anytime I was working on this book, which meant my left shoulder was somewhat tense but not burning due to over stress. The process of attempting to write a book is stressful as well as other concerns: What if no one wants to read it? What if they do buy a copy and they don't like it and ask for their money back? I am so fortunate to be able to apply the principles in this book that allow me to deal with the stress level I am dealing with currently.

A common sign of being over stressed is for someone to stop caring what happens to them or anyone else. Of course, this is also a sign of depression and could possibly be a sign of thoughts of suicide. If you know of anyone who is giving away their possessions unexpectedly, then that is more than a red flag. It is a major warning sign of suicidal thoughts!

This is one of the scariest things about being a provider who has the ability to write prescriptions is that you may have a patient who is very depressed *and* is contemplating suicide. As a caring provider you give them appropriate antidepressants, which work well enough to help them with their depression. It is very unfortunate that they now get to feeling well enough to carry out their plans to kill themselves! One question providers always have to ask is "Are you considering hurting yourself?" Often, the patient is untruthful with their answer because they don't want anyone to know their plans. Not only does the provider have to ask the question, but they have to document that they asked the question and put the patient's response in the patient's medical file. If you ask this question but fail to record it, the old adage holds true: "If you did not document it, it did not happen!" So, if the patient takes their life after seeing the provider, then the family can sue the provider, and if you did not document that you asked the question, as well as the patient's response, you could lose everything you ever worked for, including your ability to practice medicine. How's that for stress when your overwhelming desire is to help others?

Early in my career as a provider, I had a patient take their life by taking nearly all of their valium at one time. When I saw the patient, he had already been taking the valium for months as verified by his records in the prescription monitoring program that shows any controlled substance received in the last twelve months. When the police picked up the body, there was a prescription bottle with my name as the provider. He did die of an overdose and left a note of suicide in his room, and the local authorities did an investigation showing that I had not done anything inappropriate in my treatment plan. There is a great deal of stress when you are a provider that many people don't realize.

So, if anyone is now apathetic (not caring) when they seemed to care earlier, please take it as a warning sign and spend some time with them because you may very well save their life! One quick way is to observe their attention to their clothing and grooming if they were fastidious about it before. Their lack of desire to eat if they are not worried about their weight is another sign of apathy.

One of the worst things that happens when people don't care about themselves any longer is that they stop taking medications that they might need, so their physical health deteriorates quickly and sometimes irreversibly. Some of their medicines might even be for depression, and if they come off of them, it will take several days to a few weeks to notice a difference in their behavior and attitude.

Anxiety/Post Traumatic Stress Disorder (PTSD)

We all have anxiety at times and most often for justifiable reasons. My anxiety always goes up when I approach a "speed trap" while driving, even if I know I am driving just a little over the limit. There is little in life that is as humbling as to have an officer stop you. The anxiety we are concerned about in recognizing someone's stress level is when they are anxious and don't have an identifiable reason. This anxiety is ongoing, and we deal with it daily and still can't ascertain why we have the anxious feelings.

Some have very well-identified reasons for their anxiety and stress that may have been from war, military service, abuse, death of others, near-death of ourselves, serious accidents, major or chronic illness... etc. that certainly raise our stress level. We will address how to reduce and/or overcome our identified Post Traumatic Stress Disorder (PTSD).

Irritability

When you or anyone else important in your life is irritable for an extended period of time without a good reason, it is a diagnostic sign of depression and/or being over stressed. Many of us have irritable times when nothing is going right, until we wisely realize that maybe we are the one with the problem and it's not the rest of the world that is making our life miserable! Often this is a change in behavior for the person, so it can be used to help diagnose being over stressed rather than depressed.

Mental Fatigue

My definition of mental fatigue is when you sit at your workplace and nothing happens! It is as if your brain has gone into "sleep mode" when you need it, sometimes desperately, not only to stay awake but to function on all cylinders. I remember a recent mental fatigue session when I was leaving on a much-needed vacation. I had hired another provider to take my place for a week, and she came in on Friday afternoon to learn our electronic medical system (EMS). She also took four of my afternoon patients. If she had not voluntarily taken those patients, I honestly believe that my vacation would have been spent wearing one of those white jackets where you can't move your arms!

I went on vacation to one of my favorite places in the United States—Monument Valley, Utah, where I spent many years vacationing as well as ten weeks of clinicals. I was almost brain dead for the first few days but was able to recover quickly because I was able to interact with friends and witness a branding session by the Navajo where they roped the cattle and horses while the Indian "cowboys" were on foot rather than using horses. You talk about a rodeo! Fortunately, the week of vacation recharged my mental batteries, but when one is way over stressed, it may not be so.

Avoiding Things

Too much stress can cause you to avoid doing even routine chores. Some people are so stressed that they don't pay their routine bills even when they have the money. Some people at work will not do routine and important reports as they have in the past. One major avoidance is to come to work late to avoid that important requirement. One of the easiest ways to terminate an employee is to show that they are late for work even after oral and written warnings. You can save time going to a lawyer if you attempt to sue anyone who fires you for being late to work even if you might have some other situations that are litigation worthy.

One way I reduced my stress when I worked for DuPont was to avoid some reports that I could not justify. There were two different reports that I was to complete, and I did so for the first few months, as anyone would who wanted to succeed. I began to question these two reports and could not even get a straight answer about why or even to whom they were to go. So, I just stopped doing both of them, and I never heard a word about it. I had determined that if someone asked me why I had not filed them when I had before, I would start doing them again. If a report or job function is not important, your boss will be glad to drop it so you can be more efficient in what they now want you to do as a productive employee.

Going to Extremes

A sign of over stress is when we are doing just about anything to an extreme. Of course, most of us think of using some type of drug too much as our first thought in this area, and that is certainly appropriate, but we must also be aware of other areas. It may be that someone is attempting to do something so very well that they cannot let it go and move on to the next step in the process. It has to be perfect for them, when actually the recipient may be more than satisfied with what you had three revisions ago.

Administrative Problems

Problems with the administration or management are also a sign of too much stress, so managers or administrators need to be aware of this constantly. It could be that the employee is not trained adequately or is incapable of performing the job they are now responsible for. If we don't handle our stress appropriately, we can find ourselves in trouble just about anywhere in our life by failing to take care of business.

Legal Problems

When we are unduly stressed, we can get into legal difficulty faster than we ever thought. If a person is using some type of drug to compensate, there is always that risk that can stay with them for life. Automobile accidents or driving violations can creep up on you quickly and add even more stress in your life. Even not paying your routine bills can become a legal problem.

Physical Signs

There are some signs of being over stressed that are more obvious than others. Irritability and anxiety are two that can be more obvious, as can ignoring personal grooming.

Illnesses

Many family practice providers recognize that more than half of their patients' illnesses are either from undue stress or exacerbated (made worse) by stress. Tension headaches are a prime example, but even migraine headaches cause tension to the body to increase the pain level of the headache.

Frequent respiratory illnesses are another potential sign of stress. Just about any time someone is ill more frequently than the general population, we need to suspect stress as a contributing factor if not the cause.

Physical Exhaustion

My personal experience after having two children and all the physical requirements required to keep them safe, warm, and fed is that "You can't die of exhaustion!" You may wish to die or not be able to understand why you are not already dead, but it appears that exhaustion is a sure sign that your body needs rest and plenty of it.

My definition of physical exhaustion is when you awaken in the morning after several hours of sleep and you are just as tired as you were before going to sleep. This is a very frustrating position to be in, so we often resort to other means for energy to make it through the rest of the day.

Reliance on Drugs

Turning to any type of drug (legal or otherwise) is seldom a positive course of action. There are some instances where a medical provider can prescribe appropriate medications, but hopefully they are short term and you can learn to deal with your undue stress by other means and eventually reduce or eliminate the need for that medication. Fortunately, there are many excellent medications with few side effects that can benefit you for the short term.

Ailments

Some ailments are more readily identified with undue stress or a system of dealing with stress that is not adequate for your stress level. Tension headaches are the type of headache that starts later in the day and becomes worse as the day progresses. A tension headache usually starts in our head or neck and progresses all over the head and neck; often when we have pain in one part of the head or neck, we cause spasms in the neck muscles because we are attempting to hold our head very still to minimize the pain. That is why it feels so very good to relax our neck muscles or take a break. Overnight the muscles relax so that we often don't have the pain upon awakening.

Blood pressure can be negatively affected by undue stress, but it usually does not manifest as a physical symptom until your blood pressure gets high enough to cause concern about a stroke. That is why hypertension (high blood pressure) is called the "silent killer." Your body is able to accommodate the high pressure of the arterial blood for years, but then several organs begin to fail at approximately the same time. One reason a provider looks into the eyeball is so they can check for "flame hemorrhages," which are caused by high blood pressure. Also, high blood pressure is very damaging to those super thin membranes in the kidneys that separate the blood from the urine. The very fragile membranes allow material from the blood to pass through to the urine so they can be excreted. After the high blood pressure "beats up" the fragile membranes for a long time, they begin to fail and the patient goes into kidney failure just from not addressing their uncontrolled hypertension.

I had an interesting patient who was in kidney failure from uncontrolled hypertension. She was 84 years old and when I told her that I had made a referral for her to a kidney specialist, she related that she would not go. When I asked her why, she said she was 84 and was going to have to die from something, plus she was ready to go on to Heaven and not be a burden to her family. I discussed with her at length that she could live a good deal longer if she kept the appointment, but she assured me that she would not go even after I told her that her multiple laboratory results indicated kidney failure. A few months later she was in with another ailment that required her to take some mild, generic drug for a few days. She related that she was concerned about what the drug would do to her liver. My response to her was "What do you care since you are already in kidney failure and refuse to seek appropriate care!" We all had a good laugh about that, and she agreed to take this medicine.

One patient had such a serious skin condition due to stress that I was not willing to accept that as a diagnosis! This young female had what we call a "model" complexion, which is usually from one parent with darker complexion and the other with fair skin. This gives the child the hardiness of the darker skin but the youthfulness of the fair-skinned parent. She actually never even had any signs of acne as a teenager. She was extremely bright and had been identified early in her childhood as intellectually gifted. She is a member of Mensa, which is an association that is comprised of gifted individuals who score in the 98th percentile on standardized IQ (intelligent quotient) tests. She scored a 98 on two different tests and a 99 on a third test. With a percentile ranking, you cannot make 100 by definition of the method of ranking. She had expressed disappointment that she had not made 100 until I told her that a 99 was really the equivalent of 100 on other rankings. Her IQ averaged 140 over the three tests. I am telling you how intellectually gifted she was to establish that she had the brain power to deal with life's stressors because she could understand most life situations.

For about four years her skin was the worst that I had ever seen on any patient. She had open sores on most of her body that required almost continual antibiotics to keep from becoming infected. I recognized immediately, the first time I saw her, that her condition was nothing I was trained or qualified to handle, so I arranged an appointment with the same dermatologist I had used for years as a consultant, as well as personally. His assessment was a stress-related illness. I was not willing to accept that since it was so severe, so I sent her to a well-known dermatologist I had studied under when I was receiving my medical training. His diagnosis was the same, but he did greatly encourage her by telling her that the sores would not leave a scar unless she irritated them further by "picking" at them.

Now I was really concerned because I had two specialists with the same diagnosis, and the odds of them both being incorrect were very low. I still sent her to another dermatologist, who came up with the same diagnosis. The patient's fear as well as mine was that if undue stress was causing that much of a problem with her skin, what on earth was it doing to the rest of her body that was not as visible? She was on a full course of behavioral therapy at the MD level and was compliant with his medications. Her skin condition was so severe that she no longer wore any clothing that did not cover her completely for all of the four years, when she was at an age when all her friends were enjoying time at the lake or pool. Both her psychiatrist and I were concerned that her skin condition was severe enough that she would commit suicide. Neither of us would have been surprised to learn of her taking her own life due to this condition, especially when it began to manifest itself all over her body and her lovely young face.

The good news about this patient was that when she was able to reduce her stress level and learn to better deal with her life, which was very stressful due to circumstances beyond her control, her skin condition completely cleared up! And without any scarring! She began to use a self-preservation technique that will be discussed later. Even after ten years or so, she is still amazed that her skin has returned to its youthful appearance, such that most people think she is much younger than her chronological age. She had such a will to live that she overcame the thoughts of taking her life, examined her life, and eliminated or minimized the external stressors by using that wonderful brain to deal with her very stressful life. She now has a daughter and she is so thankful that she was able to overcome her stress. I call her "Mensa mom."

Stomach Upset (milk allergy)

You may be awakened at night by a feeling of nausea due to stress, but it may also be due to something as simple as a milk allergy. I used to really enjoy a very cold glass of milk (putting the glass and milk in the freezer for about fifteen minutes) and warm chocolate chip cookies. I would often awaken with nausea several hours later. One day I was discussing with a patient that they might have an allergic reaction to the milk, and it hit me that maybe I did also! I stopped drinking milk and my late night nausea went away completely, so it was not stress that was causing the problem in my case.

Humans are the only animals that drink milk as adults. In the real animal world, they all stop drinking milk when weaned and as they become more mature. I am not suggesting that you stop drinking milk, but some of your stomach upset may be from a milk allergy. Fortunately, it is easy to determine if you have a milk allergy. All you have to do is stop drinking milk or eating any dairy products for seven days to see if there is still a problem. Often you can still eat cheese even if you have a milk allergy as I found I could, after determining that milk was the culprit in my late night nausea.

Chest Pain (go to ER)

Sometimes undue stress can cause chest pain that can also be caused by or similar to an anxiety attack. Don't fool around with this one—go to the nearest emergency room as quickly as possible! Don't drive unless absolutely necessary; have someone take you or call for emergency transportation. It is far better to be told by the ER staff that you are **_not_** having a heart attack and be somewhat embarrassed than to cause irreparable damage to your wonderful heart. An untreated heart attach can cause irreversible damage to the tissue and thereby limit your lifestyle significantly even if it does not take your life. I worked for two years in the emergency department in a rural hospital and witnessed many instances where patients had delayed too long in coming to the ER. You do not die or have irreparable damage to that wonderful pump in your chest if you are experiencing a panic attack.

It is good to know the signs and symptoms of a heart attack and to also realize that many patients have had other smaller attacks but did not seek immediate medical attention. Women need to realize that the signs and symptoms for them are often not as clear cut as for men. After menopause the rate of deaths from heart attacks is approximately equal for men and women. After a heart attack the survival rate for women is less than for men. So ladies who may have already saved your male partner's life or health, make certain that you take adequate precautions and also seek immediate medical care if you even suspect you might be having an attack.

Social Withdrawal (easier now with electronics)

One common symptom of undue stress is social withdrawal, but that may not be as good an indicator now as in the recent past because people are using social media rather than interacting personally with others. It might be better to ascertain if the person is withdrawing from others *and* the use of social media. There have been predictions by sociologists that our people skills and interaction will diminish with the increased use of social media rather than just having person-to-person interaction. I have found that often even person-to-person interaction is negatively impacted by social media use, or the person allows social media to interrupt social interaction. I now have the habit of stopping talking mid-word if the other person allows their electronic device to interrupt the conversation because they are no longer listening to what you are saying due to their concern of what they might miss from the outside source.

Strategies

We have discussed a great number of areas to be aware of for ourselves and others to adequately determine if we have undue stress in our lives. I have certainly not been able to list them all or even identify everything that indicates someone is unduly stressed. Now that we recognize that we are stressed to the level that it is detrimental to our health and interactions with others, it is time to focus on what we can do about it. I assure you that everything I write about as a strategy I have tried, and most I use daily to help me deal with the super high numbers from the above Holmes and Rahe scale. If I did not use these time-proven strategies, I would already be ill or to that "no stress" level of termination of life.

This is something I have to do each and every day of my life because I need to do it for me and my family. Our world today is EXTREMELY stressful! We need to be aware of how our world today is different from any other time in history, how the stressors have increased, and how we can—and must—alter our lives to adequately deal with these troublesome times. We must protect those around us who we are responsible for and who may not be aware of their own stress level or how to deal with it even if they do realize it. One ten-year-old female child asked her mother if she could go to a counselor to help her deal with her stress. There is much to be said for the maturity of this pre-teenage or "tween" young lady to seek assistance, but it is sad that she has that much stress to deal with at that age. She is receiving adequate care now, and hopefully some of her problems will be resolved or minimized soon.

Physical Exam

One of the first items on your agenda for reducing stress is to make certain that you don't have some organic problem complicating your life. You could have a hormone imbalance, early diabetes, allergies, thyroid problem, sleep apnea...etc. Any of these, plus others, could be causing you far more problems than you can imagine until you ascertain what the problem is and how to address it. It is amazing to me personally and professionally what allergies can do to you. When you are allergic to something, it is often cumulative and unnoticed because you don't realize that you are impacted so negatively until you get to feeling better.

Allergies were a tremendous problem for me, and I will not bore you with the details, but a quick example is how they impacted my graduate education. Often I would go to the library to reduce distractions so I could focus on studying, but I would become so sleepy that I was not productive. Later when I was tested for allergies, the results indicated that I was extremely allergic to the mold that grows in books! So the library was the *last* place I needed to be studying. Often libraries have special offices you can use for privacy, but even that benefit was out for me.

I have known many very successful business people who had to overcome their allergy problems in order to succeed. One business acquaintance of mine was really struggling with his health issues. He was tested for allergies, began treatment, and is now the "big cheese" of the largest primary care organization in the entire state. He had all this natural ability to be a business leader, but his "edge" was knocked off due to the constant fatigue and other allergic symptoms keeping him from his optimum level. The first time I met this young man about 25 years ago, I was immediately impressed with him! He was one of those individuals you meet in your life that you would like to "purchase stock" in, as if they were a corporation. As a manager working for DuPont, we were well trained to look for excellent talent, and this young man was off the chart from my estimation. His success in a very difficult medical business has proven my assessment correct. If he had not sought treatment for his allergies, he may not have achieved his current level of success.

Allergy testing and treatment were certainly important in my life personally also. One of my most severe reactions was to mold. At the time I was the most ill, we found that mold was growing on the floor under our bed in the rental house we were using during graduate school. So I was spending several hours a night breathing the worst allergen for me. It was so severe that I had to withdraw for one full semester of physical-organic chemistry graduate school. I found I was sleeping all night and taking two several-hour naps per day after I withdrew from school. Then we found the problem and I was able to return to school. Even after taking allergy injections for years, I have to be careful around any mold in any hay as I feed my horse.

Allergy testing is often paid for by insurance companies. Ask your provider about your concerns because they usually have a simple list of symptoms and if you check some of them, it will probably qualify you for allergy testing. If you use over-the-counter (OTC) antihistamines, make certain you try the second-generation antihistamines to reduce drowsiness. Your pharmacist can give you advice, and many excellent medications are now generic. My personal favorite and the one I most often discuss with patients is loratadine (Claritin(R)) 10mg., one per day. The first-generation antihistamines like Benadryl(R) are so sedating they are often used as OTC meds for insomnia.

Build Support Systems

A support system is someone who can assist you in your quest to reduce your stress. You may have several people who can help, and I suggest you use them appropriately. If you do not have someone in your corner, then invest the time to develop such a relationship. Since nearly everyone is very stressed, it should not be difficult finding someone who could be of benefit. You might just discuss your stress with someone around you (if you have not already, since it seems to be a popular topic) and ask how they are coping with their stress level. If they are coping well, then you can learn from them; if they are not, then you have an opening to discuss how the two of you might work together to overcome your difficulty.

Men Are Not As Good At This As Women

It appears that women may have an easier time of building useful relationships among their friends. Sometimes men have greater difficulty admitting that we are struggling with our stress (or anything). If you are male and have difficulty discussing this with other men, just be aware that we are all in this struggle to make our lives better, so it is appropriate to let other males know that you are struggling. I use the term that life is "beating me up right now." Often your friends will be able to tell that you are struggling with something but hesitate to inquire for fear of offending you. When I was suffering from frequent migraine headaches, I would sometimes go to a social function because I felt it was important that I be there. I stopped doing that because I found there were few functions where it was really important that I be there, plus I could tell that I looked to be in such pain that it was very concerning to those who saw me. So, I did both of us a favor and stayed in bed until the pain subsided enough for me to rejoin society.

I really did not begin to develop male friendships until the last 20 years due to several factors. I had an office in my home for most of my long career in medical diagnostics and therefore was not around many men as I might have been if I had worked out of a corporate office. I enjoyed working from my home, but it did have drawbacks. My family did not hesitate to enter my office and ask for my attention when I was working, even when I would tell them I was essentially coordinating a multimillion-dollar business and, if I was in a corporate office, they would not have ready access to me. Also, I traveled a good deal in my assigned territory as well as giving seminars. Some of this travel interfered with my ability to establish male friendships.

I began to build my best male friendships when I stopped traveling so much and had a more routine schedule at home. I have a wonderful circle of male friends now who are invaluable to me! Unfortunately, one of my very best male friends passed away in 2012. He was a very real "leader" in our circle, and we all miss him greatly. I often ask these men to pray for me and my family, and they do the same to me. It is great to know that other successful men also struggle with similar problems, but if you did not know them well enough for them to share with you, you would never suspect that they had any problems. I learn a great deal from my friends and respect and admire them more than they realize. My male friends are one of my greatest blessings on this Earth, and if you men do not have the same, I want you to start investing time with others to develop these relationships.

Choose Relationships to Build

It is appropriate to choose someone to begin a friendship with that could benefit both of you. Determine what your interests are and begin to search among others who may have the same interest already or have a desire to "try something." If there is a club about your interest, you might want to target one of the newer members to the group, since they may not have had time to establish friendships already. Make some attempt to talk to the person you have decided might be a potential friend, even if they don't appear to be very open to conversation. I have found that often others are very pleased when I begin the conversation, but they were not certain enough about how their initiating a conversation might be received.

I have also found that often physically attractive men and women are very open to conversation because those blessed with physical good looks are often misperceived as "stuck up" and therefore may not appear be as open to conversation. I do suggest that you make your new friends among those of the same gender as yourself. Even though it might be more interesting to be with the opposite gender, too often others will misperceive your relationship no matter how platonic (nonsexual) it might be.

It seems that women are better at building friendships than we men are, but I want everyone to make certain that you have some positive friendships in your life. Often, friends are better for us in reducing stress than some family members. A wonderful place to make friends is wherever you might be pursuing the spiritual part of your life. While spiritual gatherings of peers are not perfect groups to join due to our human failings in that area, at least most people in the group have a common interest in things spiritual.

Spend Time (Investment Time)

If you want a friend, you will have to spend time with that person, but consider the time as an investment for you and hopefully for them. It will take some time to determine if the friendship will work or not. There is nothing wrong with refraining from going forward if you determine the friendship is not the best for you right now. Your time is valuable and so is the other person's, so it is appropriate to seek another friend if that appears to be the best investment of your time to reduce your stress. If this new friendship increases your stress, then definitely withdraw and keep seeking a positive friendship.

Quantity Time vs. Quality Time

To build any positive relationship, you need to be prepared to spend a good deal of time working on that relationship, but, again, consider your time as an investment in you and your quest to reduce your stress. Hopefully, time spent with someone you deem a potential friend will benefit them also. Our social world today is not very conducive to developing friendships, so it will require some focused effort on your part.

You don't have to spend a great deal of money to develop a positive relationship either. Many sports and entertainment require some initial investment, but walking or running does not require much, plus most of us need to exercise more. It is not negative to say to someone, "I really don't have the money right now to do this activity." Often they (or you) may have equipment to share or interesting ways to plan for fun time without laying out cash. You will know rather quickly if the relationship will be positive or is one that will pull down your positive attitude, so be prepared to change direction if it is best for you.

Like You Just Saw the Person Yesterday Even After a Long Separation

A way of knowing how wonderful it is to have a friend is to reflect on someone in your past who was an important part of your life, and how the last time you saw them it was just like yesterday. When you are in their presence, it is just like it was the day before, even though it may have been years. There is no time spent in having to *reestablish* the relationship; it is an immediate "annealing of the heart" feeling! This is the test of a true, positive friendship when the depth of the friendship is already established, and you only have to catch-up on a few details when you see this person again.

It might be good to contact some friends who were an important part of a happy time in your life because you will have some commonality to discuss. Now with modern social media options available, it is easier to contact others who have been important in your life. I would like to encourage you to attempt to contact some of those you went to high school with, because for many of us that was a happier time in our lives when we really did have a great deal of freedom and little responsibility.

If you were in the military, then stay in touch with those you served with as long as they are "good for you." If they are not going to be a positive part of your life, then at least be aware that you might be good for them but they may not be the positive relationship you need right now. Maybe after you have your stress level better controlled, you'll have the energy and resources to assist those who are struggling.

It is interesting to me that nearly *every* veteran I have seen as a patient has mentioned their military experience early in the first meeting. The reason these patients mention their military experience is because it was a positive experience for most of them. I was fortunate to have friends during the years that I would have been in the military, but my friends and I did not share such intense and dangerous time together, so we missed all that quantity time.

Often people speak of "quality" time, and that is certainly an appropriate term, but it only comes after you have spent "quantity" to get to know the person well enough that now the short time you spend with them is adequate for you. Even with our children, we cannot have quality time until we have invested a great deal of quantity time establishing those wonderful memories that bring us pleasure. These pleasant reflections can do so much to reduce our stress by conjuring up a time when we were amused and/or had a fulfilling time with a close friend.

Balance Activities

"Balance" is such a simple word but so difficult to achieve. It might be best if we were to think of it as first determining what is important in our lives. As I have presented this topic in seminars all over the United States, I have had attendees tell me after the seminar that they have never really prioritized what is important in their lives. This step is paramount in your quest for reducing stress in your life! If you have not prioritized your life, then I greatly encourage you to take reflective time to at least start working on this critical list of what is really important in your life. It may require a day of being alone and just focusing on this. My dentist, Dr. Mark Luck, does this often by taking time away from work to go alone into the mountains to make certain that his priorities are still where they need to be. If you have already accomplished this step and you feel confident in your evaluations, then it is still wise to relook at that area of your life, because sometimes the list has to change due to health, divorce, death of others, loss of job, and many other important things that happen in our lives.

I cannot say this strongly enough: Prioritizing your life is crucial to your ability to reduce the stress in your life and will allow you to go forward to achieve a longer, more fulfilled life. Now you will be focusing on what you determined (after much reflection) that is really important to you, knowing that what you are doing each and every day is allowing you to fulfill the important goal of prioritizing your life and achieving success no matter how small it is.

There are so many examples that we often overlook. One is the absolute importance of being a good parent, if you are one. They don't give out Academy awards for being a good father or mother, but they should because it is the most important responsibility you have toward your child. If you have children, at the end of every day you should be able to tell yourself that, today, I did the very best job I could at being a good parent. I was not perfect in my ability to do so, but I was perfect in my <u>desire</u> to do so. I remember my older daughter telling me one day that she was going to be a better parent than I was. My immediate response was "I sure hope so." We often beat ourselves up because we don't think we are good enough as parents, and sometimes our children will remind us that we are not the parent they would like for us to be. It is so humbling to be a parent and to know your mistakes even more than your children do. What helps me with this is that I focus on that part of my life because for me it is a very high priority. When any of us focus our energies on what is really important to us, we are "good by default." We have amazing capabilities when we focus on important tasks, and we need to tell ourselves that often, often, often.

Work Should Not Be #1—If It Is Then You Have a Problem

In your continual quest to keep your priorities on your radar screen, work is certainly a priority that should be strongly considered, but it should **not** be number one. Work is very important so we have income to live and provide for ourselves and any others in our family. Work will always let you down because satisfaction is so very difficult to achieve at work. Our boss will always want more, and too often we place even more stress on ourselves than even our management team does. If you recall from the Holmes and Rahe listing, a promotion is also stressful. The only thing more stressful than a promotion is <u>not</u> getting a promotion or recognition when you feel that you deserve it. There were times with my work at DuPont when I felt like I should have been given a certain position but then later realized that I did not really have the experience to have been successful even if I had landed that promotion.

It is amazing what a guilt trip management will sometimes put on you to accomplish some tasks. I have cancelled family vacations to accomplish some work task, only to find out later that the work that I did while missing a planned vacation was not nearly as important as I had been led to believe. One important goal for all of us is to be the very best employee we can be at all times. It is amazing what you can accomplish at work if you focus on being an excellent employee; you can rest assured that you will be rewarded no matter what level you are. Excellent employees are like gold in today's work and marketplace. So many employees spend a great deal of energy attempting to do the very least they can without being fired. Many attempt to come to work in barely awake mode and only become a productive employee some time later in the morning when they fully awaken.

As an employer I have been appalled at what employees will do while taking my money for a salary. Some of them bring their breakfast to work and eat and visit after clocking in and then feel that I am a terrible boss because I tell them they are to eat their breakfast on their own time, before they get to work. Many employees feel that as long as they are on the work site by the time their pay starts, they are doing as they should. Actually, employers expect (and justifiably so) that you are ready to actually start working when the time starts, not turning on your computer for it to warm up or after you have finished your morning beverage. Employees doing personal work, checking personal emails, looking for other jobs, playing games, checking Facebook, shopping, and perusing the latest news are just a few of the many things I have caught employees doing while I am paying them to work for me. I had one of my higher paid employees paying himself $31,000 more per year than we had agreed. Another employee, whom I was paying a higher salary than most, was asked to look into obtaining a grant so I could keep a clinic going in a medically underserved part of town. A volunteer was willing to help us in our medical mission of serving those who did not have adequate healthcare. My employee did not make a concerted effort after informing me that there was no justifiable need or money available even when I asked them to keep searching. A year later, it was announced that another medical group, which was also concerned for the medically underserved, had just received a $500,000 per year grant for ten years for a total of five million dollars. Therefore, it is now obvious that there was a justifiable need in that area and also money available.

Work is important, but it is not the most important part of life.

You never hear of anyone stating when close to death, "I wish I had spent a few more days at the office." In my work with DuPont, I was moving locations frequently. One move was from Kansas City, Missouri, to Dallas, Texas, for only ten months before I was promoted into the home office area in Wilmington, Delaware. I received a 15% promotion upon moving into Delaware, but due to tax differences, I took home $10 less per month and gave up a company car. I told my new boss in the home office, and he did not believe me, so I showed him my pay stubs from when I was living in Texas and what I was *not* making in Delaware after a significant raise in base pay. He was surprised. I told him that I could not afford any more promotions!

Four years later I was able to get off that "fast track" and move to Tennessee so my daughters could have a more normal school life. It was like a 30% raise leaving Delaware, plus I now had a company car. I have never regretted that move in my career because I felt that it was more important for my children to have a "hometown" than my having the potential of upward mobility in such a wonderful company. DuPont later paid nearly all the expenses for me to attend graduate school to earn a PhD in Health Services while working full time. The twenty-plus years that I spent working for DuPont were years that taught me so much—an education that benefited me greatly in all areas of my life—while also providing an excellent income and wonderful benefits. Much of what is in this book was learned from this excellent company. For many years they paid all my expenses to allow me to present seminars on stress management at many national, regional, and local healthcare meetings.

While I was living in Delaware for four years, I was very busy with two "venture projects." These were start-up businesses where I was able to be involved in nearly all areas with very little oversight. It gave me wonderful opportunities to learn and even make mistakes without being in a great deal of trouble. I never did make

WORK SHOULD NOT BE #1—IF IT IS THEN YOU HAVE A PROBLEM

any big mistakes that were obvious, but I knew practically every single one that I did and attempted to learn how not to repeat them. Unfortunately, I did repeat some of them, and that is always humbling when you know to do differently but are not able to accomplish your "perfect" goal.

Don't take your work home if at all possible! When I learned not to bring my work home, my stress level diminished significantly! I started working on this part of my life when I was in the home office working for DuPont while living in Delaware. I had a fifteen-minute drive to work in some of the loveliest parts of the state, including a beautiful covered bridge. I began "thought management" on my way home once I decided that the covered bridge was my business/home "thinking transition point." As I drove onto the bridge, I started making myself stop thinking business thoughts, so in the next seven to eight minutes I was nearly thinking only of family and home. It helped me a great deal because I began thinking of what a fortunate man I was to have a wife, children, and a home that was so very important to me, that they needed and deserved my full attention.

The next morning I would still think about family pleasures until I drove onto that lovely bridge on the way to work. Certainly it is impossible to thought-manage totally so that at home you do not think about work and you do not think about home issues at work, but it *is* possible (and easier than I thought) to focus *most* of your thoughts and energy on either home or work. After I began to see the benefit of this process and had it working as well as I could, with my limited ability, I was able to take the next step—leaving work behind as I walked out of the building to go home, and minimizing the work thoughts until I got into the building the next work day.

If you do not have a similar (or better) method to somewhat separate your home and work thoughts or mental energy, then I would greatly encourage you to make some effort to find a way to separate work from home/family time. (If you are single, you are a "family" of one and therefore must protect yourself.) If there is more than one person in your family, make certain you are able to assist the family with lowering their stress level by bringing a sense of peace to their lives also.

Your home space (no matter what it is—large or small, fancy or plain) should be your refuge from much of the stress that this life dumps upon us. It is imperative that you feel safe in your home and, if you do feel safe, be thankful that you are. So many people live in unsafe home situations from external forces in the neighborhood. Even worse are the unsafe relations within the home. I find it extremely difficult to adequately describe "home" just as I find it difficult to describe "love," but if where you spend most of your time eating, relaxing, bathing, and sleeping is *not* safe and comfortable, it is a stretch to call it home. I recommend that you change whatever you can in your life to have a home for restorative rest and relaxation. I really can't emphasis enough how very important it is to everyone that they have a "home." I have known (all too well) what it is to live in a house that should have been a home but never gave me the peace I needed to be successful in life. I have often wondered what I might have been able to accomplish for myself and others if I had felt like I had a real home. For over twenty years I stayed in a house, hoping it would get better, but it only became worse as the years progressed. I do not regret that I "invested" my time attempting to help my family because I can truly say that I took plenty of time focusing on what was most important to me. I blame myself for much of that situation, so I am not attempting to be overly negative about anyone else.

My home now is much more comfortable from a peace standpoint, and it truly helps me do the things that are important to me. I can come home and be at that wonderful place we call home. I get into that "home feeling" when I turn into my driveway. When I am off the street, I disconnect my seat belt as a further signal that I am now in a "safe" place. I have found this physical action helps me trigger my brain that now I am at a relaxing place where I control most of the environmental influences so I can find peace. All of this is very beneficial to me even when my life is very severely stressed. I am so very blessed to have a home that I enjoy (and it is a very modest home) and have found a means to maximize that home feeling when I am there. I hope everyone can achieve a satisfactory level of peace in their home—the rest of your daily life will not give you enough peace to compensate for a lack of peace at home.

When some of my patients tell me what they have had to deal with where they live, it absolutely crushes me. The different abuses some of us have to deal with are overwhelming at times, and that makes me appreciate my home that much more. I saw a good deal of this while working in the emergency room and often saw men who were injured by the women in their relationships. I had been told in my medical training that one of four women who came to the ER were there because of abuse. I challenged that statement during my schooling and after approximately three years working in different emergency settings found the number of abuse cases reported by women was much, much lower than that. We always reported any suspected physical abuse incident to the local police, and they came to interview the patient even if the patient did not want the police to talk to them. That was always a memorable event and did not happen on every shift even when I saw many other women who were not being abused nor had any signs and symptoms of physical abuse. I always tell anyone who is being abused that their abuser is a coward. Abusers do not abuse someone who has an equal ability to defend themselves, so anyone (even if female) who abuses someone weaker than they are, is a coward. Sometimes men will not defend themselves from women because of the fear of legal retaliation and also the fear of injuring that person. Abusers (cowards) will eventually attempt to abuse someone who is stronger than they think and they will experience the humiliation of being abused.

As a provider I am bound by law to report suspected abuse. I cannot be sued for that reporting, but I can be prosecuted if I do not report it. I have had to report a few cases in my clinic work in my own clinic, but when I worked in the ER, I always involved the MD to take over any suspected abuse situation.

I had an interesting situation when I reported a case of elder abuse. The patient was being abused by her adult son, who was living with—and off—her. I had her wait in my conference room and called the police. At the same time I had a potential provider who was talking to my practice administrator about coming to work with us. When she saw the police arrive and me take the officer into the conference room, she automatically assumed that I was in trouble and left without completing the new employee process. Actually, I am glad that potential employee left, because you cannot make that type of assumption when you are seeing patients. She would not have been fair to the patients, and it is better to know something like that up front. One MD working for me told me that my patients were "trash." I was so glad she left also. My patients were not the more affluent patients, but these were the patients I had chosen to serve. I would often tell people that if I were in healthcare to make money instead of serving the medically underserved, I would be doing Botox injections in the upscale part of town.

We have a free table at all our clinics where we provide clothing, food, and small appliances that others donate. It is amazing what wonderful items others have given to my patients! Some of my patients would have tears in their eyes as they told me about their "find" on the free table. The local Goodwill store manager called me one time to tell me that all their winter coats were on sale for two dollars. I bought about 26 coats for the free table for just over $50, and some of them were London Fog coats. All of the coats were nice enough that I would have used them myself if I had needed any of them.

If you are in a stressful living situation, do everything you can to make it a place of peace. It is not possible for you to do all the peacemaking if you live with others, but at least get as much peace as you can. It may require that things get a little worse temporarily so there can be more peace for you and others later. Look to social services if necessary to help you find a safe environment. Those services are supported by our taxes, so please don't feel that you are taking advantage of anyone. We all pay taxes on practically everything we buy, even if we don't pay a great deal of income tax. Please take the best of care of you and yours, which may require you to make some changes. If you are a parent, you must think of providing a safe haven for your children and protecting them from undue stress even if you feel that you can handle the stress.

Play

It is critical that we recognize the importance of fun in our lives! There are those good-feeling endorphins when you are having fun while playing and enjoying yourself. These are the natural good things that the body does to reward you for doing things right. Not only is it important that you play, but it is also important that the others in your life do also. Enjoying some activity is truly therapeutic for your total self and certainly brings down your stress level.

It may be interesting to you that one of the simplest tests for depression in patients is to just ask two simple questions. Have you lost pleasure in activities that previously were pleasurable for you? Do you feel blue or down most of the time? These two questions are about as good an indication for depression as some of the longer questionnaires that have been approved to indicate depression. I use the two-question measure most of the time because many of my patients have difficulty filling out even simple surveys, and their insurance—or lack of insurance—does not allow adequate time to ask all the other questions. One outcome of this simple test is that you can make lifestyle change suggestions or give a low dose of antidepressant after determining that the patient is not suffering from some organic reason for their illness. I have been so very pleasantly surprised to see the patient feeling much better in one to two months so that now they can feel good enough to make some lifestyle changes, allowing them to reduce or eliminate the medication.

Fun and play can do wonders in this area, but if a person is depressed, they will not enjoy the fun they enjoyed previously. So often you give a patient a low dose with careful screening and then when they feel better, you can move on to the next step in helping them heal.

There is a concern when you tell people to have more fun because often they will take that statement to mean that fun is what they should be seeking instead of contentment. If you focus too much on fun, you can become a danger to yourself or others because you are attempting to always get more of a "high" out of doing more and more. Soon you might be bungee-jumping off the highest bridge with only dental floss tied around your ankles!

Women, you need to be cautious that sometimes your male friends will entice you into fun activities that require more upper body strength than most women possess. Just look at YouTube under some of the "failure" compilations and often you will see women being injured because their male friends did not allow for the difference in upper body strength in the physical activity. Women are often just as brave as men, but some activities are just too difficult to do. Some examples are having a woman attempt to swing on a rope over water and then drop into the water...they may not have the physical strength to hold on safely until they are over the water. Another is when you see men enticing their female companion to fire a high-powered firearm, and the recoil is greater than their strength to compensate. I remember that my older daughter was very strong, and I treated her like a boy in most of our physical activities. She was able to hold her own with most boys until they began to develop the upper body strength which gave them an advantage over most girls. She was certainly courageous and bold, but I worried about her safety as she played so physically with her male friends.

God and Family

In our effort to prioritize what is really important, some struggle with the relationship of God and family in their priority list. It just doesn't seem fair to have such a large separation to put God with a number one and the family with the number two. I feel that they should be more like software updates of 1.1, 1.2, or 1.3 because they are all so important to many people. If your faith does not have taking care of and loving your families as a very high priority, then find one that does.

Family is so very important to you that is difficult to quantify the positive impact of having one and the negative impact of not having a family. I remember one day when my wife and I were flying somewhere and prior to boarding a young lady told us that she had only come to Knoxville to identify her parents, who had been killed in a motor vehicle accident (MVA) while vacationing in the Knoxville area. We asked if she had any siblings, and she said that she had no other close family members because her parents were from very small families, and death had taken most of them. I asked if she had anyone to greet her when she returned to her home city or to be with the next few days, and she said she did not. As we were exiting the plane, I stopped to tell her how much we were thinking of her, and she was genuinely pleased. We had a short time to visit due to flight arrangements, so I did not get her name and address. After returning from my trip, I contacted the local newspaper to see if I could find out her family's information but was not successful. I can only imagine what it must have been for her to lose the only family she had left on Earth, with no close friends to help her during this stressful time.

I often hear others quote, "If you have your health, you have everything!" Actually, I sincerely believe that if you have God, family, and friends, then you have everything because they can help tremendously in dealing with any health issues you might have. There are some who walk away from family without any real reason, and that is everyone's loss. There is something about that family history that makes most family interactions pleasant. If you are blessed with a good family, then please let them know as often as possible because they are invaluable!

I have been close friends with two very wealthy men who do not live in my town. One I still talk to almost every Saturday, and it is a highlight of my week. I have known him for over thirty years, and now his family has turned against him and is attempting to take everything they can from him because they don't want to wait for their inheritance. He has been extremely generous with them all their lives, but now they want more. The other man was so wealthy that when his wife divorced him, he paid her $56 million dollars and still kept all his properties and businesses. Most of his problems as he related to me were dealing with his family even after he made all of them millionaires. It is a shame that these two good friends of mine have been blessed with financial success by their hard work, but are not appreciated by those who should be the most important to them and have years of pleasant interactions instead of the friction that has driven them apart. I personally have never had enough money for my family to fight over, but I do remember how disappointed some of them were when I told them I had significantly reduced my life insurance when I stopped having other business ventures that required me to carry more life insurance. It was almost as if I had taken the money from them. I am not convinced that it is best to be worth more dead than alive!

So focus on that family, see that they are knowledgeable about spiritual matters as you rear them, even if later they don't seem to care as much as you might about spiritual matters. At least you have exposed and educated them about that important part of their lives in a similar way that we expose them to music and sports to allow them to experience the other important areas of their upbringing—later if they choose not to play a certain sport or instrument, you can feel good that you made arrangements for them to have a knowledge base from which they can make their decision.

Sometimes it is a temptation to be less kind to our families than we are to our other peers. We might not feel that we have to say please and thank you to our family as we might to others. Truly, if there is anyone you should be kind to (actually it is best to be kind to everyone), it should certainly be your family. They will not be perfect as family members maybe, but still family is so very important to you and will become more so as you mature. So please be gracious to your family and support them often. You will seldom regret doing so, but you very well may regret not being as good to them as you can.

Hobby

I feel that a working definition of a hobby is something that you enjoy doing for several hours, but it seems just like minutes have passed because you were so absorbed in something you like. This is a GREAT stress releaser! It is amazing to me how many different hobby activities there are and how many people participate in them. Often they are well organized with national conventions and club publications. This area of your life is another good way to make friends. A hobby can be very beneficial if the entire family enjoys the same activity. That is not always possible, but it is an excellent investment of your time to attempt several different hobbies, for all the family or even yourself, until you find one that makes time fly. Often a hobby can become a business, and in this economically troubled world, that could be a good thing.

I have several hobbies and they serve me well. Reading is a big one for me. A vacation for me nearly always needs to include significant reading time. I always take books with me even when I go horseback riding. I am blessed to have my own horse for riding, but while he may be able to go all day, I cannot. I have even learned to combine horseback riding with hiking. I call it "horseback hiking," and it works out so well for me. I have comfortable boots to ride and walk in, so I usually hike about 20% of the time. This gives the horse a break if he needs one; it allows me to understand better how steep some of the hills we are climbing, keeps me warmer in cold weather, and keeps me from having such muscle soreness after a long day's ride. I take many people riding with me and have for many years. I encourage all of them to get down and walk some, but often they don't and regret it later...especially the next day or so. When you ride a horse you use different muscles, or at least they are in different positions than when walking, so walking allows me to enjoy my ride more and for a longer period. Then it is back to eat, read, and rest. One time my sister brought me a bag with six books inside all by the same author just before I went on a six-day vacation. I read a book a day and still had plenty of time to enjoy the other activities on my vacation. It was one of my better vacations due to the interesting books to consume and the private time to do so.

How to Balance

Increase Energy

Since we are getting beat up by our stress, it would be great to increase our energy but only if we could manage our stress level where we are now. If we are successful in gaining more energy and we just take on more stressful parts of our life, we are no better off! There are well-proven ways to increase our energy, which we will discuss, that don't necessarily cost more money. I encourage everyone to get a physical because some of your inability to deal with undue stress may be because of a possible organic problem with your wonderful body that normally functions exceptionally well. If some of your hormone levels (male and female) are abnormal, they can significantly impact your ability to function on a daily basis. Men are not as aware of how a low testosterone level can affect them, and/or they have difficulty asking a provider about it for fear of being judged less masculine. Often providers fail to ask those important questions also, as I failed to do too often in my practice. It may be of interest that every male patient I treated for low testosterone was very "macho" appearing. I did not have any patients who had less than full masculine characteristics. These hormone levels can affect any of us at any time, and they are not always recognized until we have appropriate body fluids submitted for clinical laboratory analysis. Laboratory testing is very sophisticated and accurate today with our more modern laboratory techniques, so your confidence in the results can be higher than before. We will be discussing specific examples of how to increase energy later, but we need to establish that we also must focus on how to deal with our stress before we concern ourselves too greatly about energy gain.

Increase Success

One of the most damaging aspects of our media-focused lives is that we too often feel inadequate compared to others because they seem so successful. I personally would be more interested in a show on "Homes of the Not-So Famous" to see how others live normal lives, because most of the media darlings do NOT live normal lives, and they would be the first to admit it. It is so wonderful to be able to go out anywhere without someone taking pictures of you to sell to our media "sensationalism" society. It would also be terrible to have to hire bodyguards to protect you and your family from others. It is great not being famous, and it is something that most people desire. It is wonderful to be recognized and appreciated for your efforts, but if the media determines that they can make money off your notoriety, then it is a negative place to be. Unfortunately, once you gain that notoriety, it is not really possible to return to a more normal life because they will want any sort of news about you (good or bad) to enable them to make money.

So, please consider your future if you are thinking of gaining much recognition because there are definitive drawbacks. I actually enjoy driving around and looking at modest homes (as I have) and wondering what type of life that person has and how it would be exhibited in their home. When I am invited to anyone's home who has children, I am always desirous of seeing the children's rooms to see what they like best. My twelve-year-old granddaughter has each of her four walls painted a different color. She chose the colors very carefully and enjoys having the different colors around her. It is so interesting to meet people who are not famous because often famous people believe their own press and have a tendency to feel that they are privileged above others.

Too often we don't realize that we are *already* successful! We compare ourselves with the media magnets and think, *since I don't have what they have, I am not successful*. That is a very damaging concept and an extremely stressful situation to be in. Out of the millions of people in the United States, so few are truly famous, and often we hear so much about them that we soon tire of hearing anything else about them. We get to the point that we are *not* concerned that they are having a baby, getting married, or even getting a divorce. We should look at ourselves to determine if we are successful, and there are many ways to judge that concept. One advantage I have as a provider is that it makes me so thankful every day that I am not as ill as most of the patients who come to see me. Some of their ailments are self-inflicted, by not taking good care of themselves, but some are very ill or handicapped by no fault of their own. If you have good health and continue to work to maintain your good health, then you are successful in the healthcare world.

If you have a good job and are a good worker, you are successful. Even if the company has to eliminate your position, at least they will regret it because you were a good employee. Some of my most stressful moments have been when I have had to tell employees that their position has been eliminated. Losing a job right now is very difficult, so you want to be successful enough at your job to be able to keep it going even if the promotions seem to be so far apart. I found that sharing any good idea was often beneficial to my employment. I never was concerned that someone else would lay claim to my good ideas or suggestions. I don't know of any time in my career when someone else attempted to "steal" any of my ideas. If you are concerned that might happen, just put it in writing and keep a dated copy. One thing I learned years ago when I had one of the worst bosses of my entire career is that when he asked me to write him a memo about something, I would always start the memo with "This memo is in response to your request to write a memo about..." Therefore he was never able to use anything like that against me. I actually had to work for this man on three different occasions until DuPont finally fired him. Every time I got a promotion, it seemed he would also until they finally determined that he would not change and it was best for him to move on.

If you are a good spouse, friend, girlfriend, boyfriend, parent, then you are successful in the most important relationships in your life. That is quite an accomplishment. Many people struggle with their personal relationships and therefore feel they are unsuccessful. You don't have to have many friends to be successful in the friendship area of your life. I often ask people how long they have been married. When the number of years is several decades, I then ask if it is to the same spouse. If they say yes, I love to say that there are many people with the same number of years, but it took three marriages to equal the same number of years! They are usually amused by that, and it gives them an opportunity to discuss why (and how) they have been able to be successful in their marriage.

I feel that some of our "market-driven" holidays are very stressful, especially Valentine's Day if you have a special love in your life. Even if you are treating your special person very well with treats or unique occasions, they still feel a strong obligation to perform on Valentine's Day. When I was working in the ER, I remember the nursing staff talking about who had received the biggest and most expensive flower arrangement in the entire hospital. It was a terrible contest where everyone lost except the florist. Roses basically double or triple in cost near Valentine's Day, so a hardworking spouse who loves their spouse dearly may not be able to afford the expensive bouquet. Other special occasions can be very stressful also to a relationship like birthdays, anniversaries, Mother's and Father's Day,

Christmas, etc. These occasions should be wonderful and stress relieving rather than stress producing.

Success should not be measured by how much money you make either. I assure you that money will NOT make you happy even if there are such sayings to the contrary. I remember when I moved from the DuPont home office in Wilmington, Delaware, where the housing market was very expensive compared to Tennessee, where you received much more value for the same amount of money. This larger home impressed my "country" grandmother so much she suggested (she was never shy about interjecting her thoughts and desires on anyone) that we buy her a color TV for Christmas. I replied that she had several grandchildren, and I would be willing to contribute to the purchase of a more modern TV but not pay for all of it. She related that since I had such a big house now, I should get her one. I don't know what happened about all of that, but I did not get involved with the total purchase because of her asking for it... and she was one of my favorites of our family.

I have been blessed with some very wealthy friends, and they have been excellent relationships, but I also know how their success with money brought them many troubles. Fame was one of them—family attempting to have them declared mentally incompetent, stealing from them, and continuing to expect financial support for years after reaching adulthood. In the state of Delaware one of the big status symbols is to have a low number auto license tag. In this state if you have a low number, the plate has a black background with white lettering versus the green background with beige lettering. Just to give you an example of the money involved, just a few years ago my friend sold the "black 17" for $75,000 to an agent who was buying it for someone else who was willing to pay that plus the agent's fee of approximately 10%. This was just for the tag...not the car. In the early 1980s he sold the "black 5" for $20,000 that he had paid $5,000 for a few years earlier. The "real look" in Delaware is to have a very low black tag number on an older Mercedes-Benz rather than a newer car so it makes it appear that you are "old money" and might even be a DuPont family member. Delaware is such a small state that it has two U.S. senators and only one U.S. representative because it only has three counties. When I lived in Delaware approximately 10% of the state population worked for DuPont, and 25% of the total salaries were from DuPont.

The reason I am relating all of this is to let you know that I was not necessarily "a mover and a shaker" in the DuPont hierarchy! I did have an excellent job, but since this was the home office and I had just arrived, I was very low on the organizational chart. I found out later that I was on the fast track for promotion to greater responsibilities but not until much later. This was an important time in my life because I was comparing myself to those who were above me on the organizational chart all the way to the president of the company. That was not a good thing to do, so I began to realize that I had already achieved some level of success by just having a job and moving to the home office, even if I was a "rookie." I soon assimilated the understanding that I was dealing with very successful people so I had better behave accordingly. This was a million-dollar business education in my opinion. I was able to learn so very much about corporate America, how to work on enhancing my people skills and how to perform in business. DuPont was very strong on treating other employees with tremendous dignity. If you were a manager and had a business goal and people working for you, it was much more important that you treated your employees appropriately than to achieve your business goal. If you achieved your business goal but were not a good manager of the people who worked for you, your career would stagnate or you could even be demoted.

I realized that success was not measured by where you are on the organizational chart of any company. Just because you report to someone else does not mean you are less than that person. Even if they think they are better than you, usually they do not last long with that attitude. But they can make your work time miserable until they, or you, move to a different position. I learned to measure my success by what was expected of me and by performing to the best of my ability, not comparing myself to how well others were doing.

I had a rather high-level manager travel with me for a day who was not even in my division. I asked him how he had moved up so quickly, and he related that much of it was "chance" in that he just happened to have excellent managers who pushed for him to be successful and gain promotions. Unfortunately, that did not happen to me often enough because the same manager who was so bad while I was in Texas for ten months was my manager twice in the home office! He certainly did not attempt to promote me and was detrimental to my career. One time when I was working for him, his manager called me in to tell me that they realized *he* was the problem; they had a very nice promotion for me, but it would take about three months to move different people around so I could have this excellent position. Those three months were the worst and most stressful time of my entire time with DuPont because I had nothing to do! You would think that would be wonderful, but it was more painful than I could have ever imagined. I attended many educational seminars during those three months that actually helped me with my personal stress management quest.

I will share one occasion where it appeared that I was much higher in the company than I really was. I was a product manager with our newest model of our very successful automated clinical laboratory analyzer. This instrument concept lasted for well over thirty years in the hospital clinical labs and was one of the most successful clinical instruments ever made and sold. If a hospital bought our instrument, they had to use our specially designed chemical packs to achieve the extensive list of chemical analysis it could perform. That was a real advantage to DuPont because we had a revenue stream after selling the equipment, but since clients could only get their reagents from DuPont when something went wrong, they could not use another product. My job required that I see about launching this product and keeping the reagent stream viable. One day one of the reagents had some problem, and I asked for a meeting with manufacturing to see what we could do about it. Manufacturing called us "corporate" people many things, but openly they referred to us as "suits." I had toured the manufacturing facility but had not had any meetings there. When I requested the meeting with manufacturing, I expected only a few people to be in attendance. When I arrived I was the only "suit," and there were about twenty people around this big conference table! I thought there must be some mistake because I had absolutely no authority over manufacturing, so I could not call any meeting but had to ask politely if we could have one. Anyway, they put me at the head of the table, and they were looking at me like "Who is this guy?" Their initial questions indicated what they thought of me, and I was beginning to wonder what I had gotten myself into by asking for a simple meeting about this important product and them treating it with their major resources. After ten minutes into this very uncomfortable session, one of the upper level manufacturing managers came to interrupt the meeting to tell me that I had a phone call. Everyone was looking to see how I was going to handle this interruption of "their" meeting. I asked him to get the name and number and I would call them back, which is exactly the correct response in that situation, I think.

The manager said, "You probably want to take this call now" because it was from one of the top guys in DuPont and one I had never even met. He named this person loudly enough that everyone could hear, because even he was impressed that this man would be calling for me. I was NOT impressed; I was scared totally to death. I thought this was the end of my short career in the home office. When I did go to the phone, it was a minor call, and if this upper level manager had realized that twenty of his employees were sitting there waiting on me, he would not have called, or he would have been very satisfied for me to call him back. This whole scenario was just like out of a movie! When I came back to the conference room, I think they were even surprised that I did come back. I sat down without telling anyone what the phone call was about, because if I had told them, they would have said he should not have interrupted us for that trivial item in our business world! What was amazing was how the "personality" of the meeting changed. Now they were fully cooperative, and we moved forward, and *they* actually solved the problem quickly.

Another time when I was given temporary power that would have taken me thirty years to achieve was when I was on another new product program. Since this was a new product and was not bringing in the many millions of dollars as my other product, it was certainly not a high priority for manufacturing. I even suspected that some of the manufacturing folks were some that the other divisions did not want. In corporate lingo it is called "dressing a turkey up to look like a peacock" and moving them to some other group so they would have to deal with them. I related earlier that I had no authority over manufacturing, and they were doing the shipping of our product's disposables, which was our revenue stream. So, I invited the overall manager of all the businesses that I dealt with to a presentation of our marketing team so he could see where we were doing well or needed to improve as well as inform him of the shipping problem. I had seven sales representatives across the U.S., so I asked each of them to come to the home office for a one-day meeting to give a 20-minute presentation on what we were doing correctly and what we needed to change to be more successful. Actually, this was quite a project to get such a high-ranking manager to commit for most of a day and to have employees travel from as far away as California to Delaware for a one-day meeting.

The meeting accomplished my goal totally, but in a way that I did not expect. The first three presenters of the status of their sales territory and problems were basically the same. Most things were going well, but the biggest problem was that after they made the sale for the equipment, we had a great deal of difficulty getting the disposables to the customers who were so excited about using this new technology. It was mid-morning by the time the third presenter was finished, and we took a short break to plan lunch selections for the group. The manager, who was about five notches above me on the organizational chart, called me aside. He said it was obvious that things were going well except for the shipping problem. He said, "I want you to make this a high priority to make this shipping problem no longer a problem." I replied that I would start working on it the very first thing in the morning after the staff had completed their presentations and returned home. I was so very pleased that he had made this a high priority!

I was not aware of how high a priority he had made it until he said, "I don't want you to wait until tomorrow to start working on this problem." I replied that I had flown the staff from all across the U.S. and felt an obligation to hear their presentations. He replied that he felt the other presentations would be very similar and that he wanted me to leave the meeting, go to the manufacturing plant, have the entire disposable product moved from the manufacturing area, and have the properly organized shipping completely set up by the end of the day! I thought this would take me weeks to set up meetings with the right people at both manufacturing and shipping to get all the necessary protocols approved and in place, and he wanted it done in basically half a day!

Actually, I like making things happen, and have done that chore for most of my life. I love a challenge to bring several people together on something and put it into place, and I felt comfortable doing that, but I never would push so many people to do anything on such short notice when they had no idea I was even coming to the manufacturing plant. This situation was a classic "talk softly and carry a big stick." I went to manufacturing without even being certain who the responsible person would be to make the decision to move the product to the shipping facility. Every person I saw that day told me that they would work on it soon, but it could not be done that day, and I could tell that I was ruffling many feathers by even requesting anything—not only was I a "suit," but I was suggesting an impossible timeframe. I used the same technique several times that day. I said I understood what a difficult problem I was causing for them, but if we could not make this happen today, they would need to explain to this manager why we were not successful in achieving the unreasonable goal. After manufacturing agreed to take the product to our shipping facility in their personal vehicle that afternoon, I had to go to shipping to get them to agree to accept this totally new product and take it on as their responsibility. I met the same resistance, but the technique worked so well that I began to wish I had the same clout as the manager who sent me so I could *really* make things happen. By the end of the day, I was able to inform him that everything was in place to start shipping the very next morning. The staff was so relieved to know that now the shipping problem was solved.

Needless to say the very next morning, I was back to my position of no authority over manufacturing, but it seemed that everyone at manufacturing remembered me from what happened that special day. I did feel that I was now viewed in a different light by the manufacturing personnel even if I no longer had the temporary authority of the upper-level manager. As a product manager in the DuPont Company, you had tremendous responsibility and almost no authority, and this was by design. This was a true learning experience for anyone who wanted to move up in the company. Just about anyone could make things happen if you had the authority to tell others what to do, but to be able to interact with "non-reports" (those who did not work directly for you) and still accomplish your goals was certainly a very important part of on-the-job education! I would often get calls from other companies asking me to come to work for them as a product manager (I am confident that they contacted everyone in every company with the same title). I would ask what the responsibilities were for this new offer, and most often it was overseeing the literature for the product or shipping or pricing as a total job, so I would just say no because at DuPont we had the responsibility for *all* of that already. The year or so that I worked in this role taught me so much about how to deal with others, to get my goals accomplished without stressing the other person out so much that they made the entire process difficult. While I had some unique experiences, most of the time I was on my own. I was so blessed to learn better how to appreciate others and their agendas and not just to look after my own agenda.

Wherever you are in your career, you are successful if you can keep a job or even get a job, because no one is going to hire you if they don't feel that you are already what they want and will grow to handle more responsibility. One of your stressors right now might be that you recognize that you are not doing the very best job you can where you work, or as a mother, or as a friend. It is so stress-relieving to be able to tell yourself that you know you are doing the very best job you can even if others do not realize it. If they do not realize your contribution now, they will at some time because any employer knows the value of a good employee.

When I have not performed well with some managers, I go to them and say, "I don't feel I have been the employee I would like to be." Then I ask them if they would help me do better. I have been absolutely amazed at the positive reaction to my admission and for seeking their advice. Even in the business world this is not seen as a weakness but a mature assessment of a problem and asking upper management for their advice. Every time I did this, we had a frank and open discussion about what I thought the problem was, and we worked together to make *me* better. I also went away feeling better about my manager. If you need to do something similar, I would greatly encourage you to do so quickly. We spend too many hours at work to have most of it stressful. Work always has an element of stress, if for no other reason than you know you have to perform or you will be out of a job.

Work allows us to provide for ourselves and our families, so it helps to see it as a positive part of our lives; it brings rewards (in the form of money) to show we are valued by our employer because otherwise they would not allocate money for our position. You are valuable as an employee and you want to bring the most value to the table every day. When you know in your heart of hearts that you are doing a good job, there is a peace that can help you be less stressed. No one is giving you this money. You are earning every penny of it, and you can take pride in the fact that someone realizes your worth (in dollars) to the business.

When I was selling large clinical instruments to some of the smaller hospitals, it was so amazing to find that often I was being paid more than the administrator, or at least my benefit package of salary, car, expense account, etc. was equal to his or her income. This realization allowed me to approach them as an equal rather than as someone who was unworthy of their time or signature authorizing a multi-year commitment to buy a great deal from our company. When I shared this with my peers at a regional meeting, they began to incorporate this "equivalence" feeling as they dealt with those who they perceived as "higher." It helped us all to do better in placing this equipment.

Never, ever think you are better than anyone on earth, but also have an equal feeling and assurance that you are no less than anyone on this planet. This is so helpful in dealing with others. When you know *internally* that you are as important as anyone, then you can much more easily deal with those who might feel more important than they really are. In my seminars I often talked to other seminar presenters who kept "score" with how big the audience was. I was fortunate not to get caught up in that scorekeeping early in my speaking career when I realized the smaller groups were more conducive to interaction with the audience, thereby increasing everyone's pleasure. If there are hundreds of people in the audience, you can only see the first few rows, so you feel like you are talking to a dark room for the most part. That is why often at concerts they will turn the lights up and have the spotlights scan the crowd so the performers will gain a perspective on how many people are there beyond the first few rows.

What's Really Important?

Always keep a running, fresh evaluation of what is really important in your life and focus on that list. Often we employees can lose our proper perspective and put business success ahead of other things (and relationships) that are far more important. Others may be impressed with the work you are doing, if that is important to you, but later in your life when you retire, very few are impressed with what you did before you retired. Later in your life, your career may not be as fulfilling as you had hoped, so work on prioritizing your relationships that will continue until you really "retire" from this earth and are "pushing up daisies." Hopefully others will regret your final termination, but others may welcome your demise. That is a difficult feeling, but just about everyone has someone, somewhere, who does not like them. I had an excellent employee who had a wonderful personality. She and I used to discuss how for much of our lives we felt that everyone liked us, and how we were devastated when we first realized that there were others who did not like us. I don't remember what incident caused her to come to this important revelation, but I can easily remember mine. It was as early as high school when I had someone tell me that they didn't like me, at first. That was a shock to me because I hardly knew this person and certainly could not remember any interaction to cause them to dislike me that I knew of. When I recovered enough to ask them why, they related that they didn't like the way I walked. I was incredulous! I could not believe that anyone would make that decision about another person just by their normal gait.

We do judge others incorrectly some of the time, but most often we are correct in our assessment of others because we have been doing it for so many years. We are often correct enough that we sometimes think we cannot make a mistake. So while you are working on realizing that you are important, just remember that others are also, and you can easily misjudge others. Once you feel that you are always correct in judging others, it will begin to impact your relationships negatively. I even had someone tell me that they knew what I was thinking! How arrogant is that? When this person told me that, I began to laugh and told them that in the future I did not need to talk to them because they could just read my mind. Others have said that they can think so much faster than others can talk, as if they are the only ones who can do that. Everyone can think faster than others can talk unless they are on medication or have an illness that slows down their brain function.

What Happens/Worst Case?

We are often stressed by "imaginary" concerns. We are so worried in this day and time, and much of it is due to our media's "addiction to sensationalism" reporting. With our wonderful advances in communication, we are able to know the worst of what is happening worldwide almost as soon as it happens. Not only are we informed about the negativism once, but it goes on for days and days if the media deems it of monetary worth. There are millions and millions of people on this earth who have nothing happen to them every day for most of their lives, but the media (which has such power to do good) focuses mostly on the negative and then throws in our faces for days afterward. This is killing us from fear!

There are many *real* reasons to be concerned, but our constant exposure to negativism causes us undue stress and worry. The **NEWS** (**N**orth, **E**ast, **W**est, and **South**) is really not "the news," it is the **bad news!** An example is of how many are fearful of flying based on hearing and seeing all the carnage of an airplane crash (which is terrible, if you are on the flight), but the media never mentions that air travel is the safest way to travel. Driving is far more dangerous than flying, but the "disaster" reports never mention the low percentage of lives lost flying after detailing the latest airline disaster. And then on top of that negative news, they list the last several plane crashes over the last several years. They retell the stories of crashes that we already knew about and did not need to be reminded about again.

How many times did you watch the towers fall in New York City on 9/11/2001? Once was enough! I am so amazed that only 3,000 were killed that day when the death rate could have been ten to fifteen times as many. That was a horrible incident, but to see it over and over with every negative detail (even in slow motion) just drives that negative picture deeper into our brain. Once is all we need to see any disaster, and even with that viewing we need to keep it in perspective regarding the millions of times the same does *not* happen. Unfortunately, there are some very evil, criminal, sick people in this world, but fortunately, there are very few of them.

If we are stressed by worry about something in our lives, it really does help to ask ourselves what truly happens if the worst case does come to be, as well as what are the odds of it even happening in the first place. One thing that has really helped me in my medical training is that if you are okay with your own death, then you can deal better with the death of others. That has helped me tremendously! We are all going to die sometime, and if we are confident in our preparation for the future, we can rest much better and reduce our stress level tremendously. We should provide for our family the best that we can, of course, but even in this case they can often care for themselves better than we might think.

I mentioned earlier how high my stress level is at this time in my life, but this "worst case" technique has eased my stress greatly. If I don't worry about my death, then it gives me a freedom for the future, which is very difficult to explain but a wonder to experience. I am concerned about a home invasion partly due to the work I do—because criminals might think I have narcotics at my home (I don't even have them at the office)—but I keep my doors locked, have motion detector lights at night, and have an adequate burglar alarm and protection if someone were to enter my home unlawfully. I would never shoot anyone for stealing anything I have, because anything they want could be replaced. They would not be interested in the things that mean so much to me, like pictures. If I were home alone I would not even leave my bedroom. I would yell or even fire into the ceiling to scare them off rather than have a physical confrontation with anyone who could cause me bodily harm or the pain of doing physical damage to them over what little I choose to have. Now, if any one of my family were here at home, I would confront them without regard for my safety or any physical damage that might come to the criminal invader. If they were to come into my bedroom, I would shoot to kill because they would only be there with the intent to harm me. I have an obligation to protect myself because I am also responsible for protecting my family and to help others with my medical training to assist in serving the medically underserved.

Parents need to know that some of your freedoms are diminished when you have the responsibility of taking care of your children. We must protect ourselves because no one on this earth will (or can) take care of your children as you can. They deserve all of you.

Over my long life I have known of many, many people to lose their jobs. Nearly all of them have told me later that they are now better off and more content than before. Often they say they wish they had been fired earlier. I have never known any of them to starve to death or be unable to take care of their family. Few have even had to move from their current home unless their new job requires a move.

We have tremendously resilient bodies and productive lives to help us deal with problems, if we need to, so we need to have confidence in ourselves that we can handle whatever happens whenever it happens. I remember my father-in-law telling me that we young people could not make it if we were faced with the same situations as he was. I quickly replied, "If you could make it, then we could make it!"

Just Say NO!

The wonderful concept of "just saying NO!" is very difficult for me. I default to "yes" when just about anyone asks me anything because I have this inherent desire to help others. This has caused me to make some poor judgment calls in my life. I sincerely enjoy helping others, so this is something I have to work on, often.

It is better to have a reason when you say no to a request even if it is a perceived honor to be asked. The one that works best for me is "I have so much to do right now that I would not be able to put forth a good effort on your project and I don't want to disappoint either of us." That is not an untrue statement because I do have a great deal of other things to do in my life. If the person is persistent, I may say, "I really will fail you because this is not now, nor will it ever be, high on my priority list." I have found that they always find someone else, and I am confident that person has done a better job than I would have.

I used to take every offer to help others in any way that I could, but even as much as I enjoy helping others, it is not good for my stress level to say yes when I should say no. I am stressed when I don't have something to do that helps others. But I realize that I cannot do all that needs doing in this world, or even in my knowledge base of my home area. A few times the requestor has attempted to use the "God will not be pleased" mentality when I say no. I found this response started working well the first time I used it: "I am so pleased that **YOU** have such a good relationship with God because if He discusses His displeasure about my refusal with you, then you are close enough to Him to smooth it over and save me from His retaliation."

Just remember, it is okay to say no. You will find that your life goes on (often better), and the "super important" job will get done without you. It is a method of helping you focus on your most important priorities and not attempting to help everyone with their important priorities.

Increase Energy

One of the very best ways to deal with stress is to increase your "real" energy. We have just discussed the need to say no, and that is important to remember as we discuss this topic. If you are successful in increasing your energy level, but you keep taking on more and more, then you will finally get back to where you are right now on your stress level. The best way is to focus on your priorities and not the priorities of others until you can severely reduce your stress level to compensate for your own life's struggles.

A "real" energy increase is one that is within the capacity of your physical body already and not stimulants, which we will discuss later. Our society today is leading us down a path of early destruction of this wonderful body we have. Undue stress is a poison that we need to minimize and bring it into a more positive part of our lives. Even our media is destructive to our bodies because the advertisements pay the media expenses. The advertisements can cause physical damage by attempting to convince us that it is abnormal not to have a bowel movement every day. For some, that is their normal routine, but for many others it is not. Many patients of mine have gone to dangerous extremes to achieve something that may not be their body's normal routine.

The advertisements also make us feel worse about ourselves because we don't look like some media sensation. I remember always wondering why the shirts on the male models in the clothing magazines seemed to fit so very well. One time I was in San Francisco and they were doing a fashion shoot in Jackson Square.

The male model's shirt fit perfectly from the front, but when he turned around during the shooting, there were many clothespins in the back holding the shirt in perfect place for the front! I was quite amused at that and have always felt better that my shirts are loose at my waist.

Exercise

You could read a hundred medical articles and as many medical books about the best way to deal with stress, depression, anxiety, weight loss, et cetera, and all of them would suggest exercise as **THE** number one thing to do. Again here I ask you to do this for yourself and not rely on someone else to notice how much better you look because you will never get enough kudos or positive input from others to motivate you to exercise.

I have heard all my life that "confession is good for the soul," and I have a confession to make.

I hate exercise!!!

Actually, in reality,

I would almost rather bleed than sweat!

I am so sorry if I have disappointed you in my confession or given you a new excuse for not exercising. Stress and depression from stress can actually keep you from having the desire to exercise no matter what you might gain. When I see patients who are depressed, we always discuss exercise, and I usually go ahead and put them on mild antidepressant medication so they will feel good enough about themselves to begin an exercise program, with the agreed-to goal of coming off the medication when they have a well-established exercise program.

I used to run and was very fortunate in that within a week or so I could run for several miles without stopping. I was never injured running, nor did I cause any damage to my body as many runners do, and that may be due to my not running as hard as they do. Ten miles was the longest distance of any organized run that I made, but I have run a few miles more than that. I have run in many of the larger cities in the U.S. in my travels. I love going out for a run early in the morning as the city wakes up because it allows such a different view of the happenings of the city.

I stopped running several years ago because even while I knew I was helping myself greatly, I was only doing that for me and not really benefiting anyone else. I am so very blessed to have two farmers living next to me who keep my horse for free. So, I decided that I would start exercising by helping them with anything physical that they would find beneficial and that was within my ability to do. For several years now I have been cleaning out fence-rows and anything else that needs cutting, hauling, and stacking to help the farmers. I don't use any power saws but cut even the big stuff with a small hand saw. That is wonderful exercise and, unfortunately, I often work up a sweat, but the benefit is worth it. The good thing about this type of exercise, for me, is that now I can look back at my work and "see" that I have done something for someone, that is so good to me, rather than just run down the road and back. I am also very blessed to live in an area that has many safe and wonderful running trails but now I mostly walk them. I visited a medical museum in Cleveland, Ohio that was a part of the Cleveland Clinic that had a display of the pressure on the heel when you run versus walking. The pressure was approximately 150 pounds per square inch with walking and about 450 pounds per square inch when running to the best of my remembrance. Whatever the actual numbers were the difference was enough for me to consider other forms of exercise even if I had never injured myself running.

2 to 1 payback

I have never felt the "runner's high" except one time when I was running in San Francisco and I felt that when I ran by a place that I had had a very pleasant visit with a good friend at the end of one of the piers. So I am not certain that the high was from the run but really from the memory of the previous evening's visit. I might run more if I had felt the runner's high but I like my current exercise routine because I can look at the work I have done with some satisfaction.

I have found on many occasions the long-term benefit is a two-to-one payback on my "investment" of time exercising. If I exercise an hour a day I can easily demonstrate to myself that I usually get an additional two hours of productive time so the net gain in, just time, and is an extra hour of productive time each day of exercising. One that is also obvious to me is that if I exercise one day and miss the next day for some reason that I still feel the extra energy until about noon the next day which would mean an approximate 18 hour "good feeling" from the exercise.

In addition to the above there are so many advantages of exercising you would think it would just be second nature to all of us. The benefits of exercise are only obvious after you have done it enough that it no longer causes soreness enough for you to wish you had not "worked out." It is amazing to me that others don't see the benefits of exercise just as much as society does not seem to realize the benefits of breast feeding! We humans are so arrogant to think we can duplicate through chemistry (remember that I am a chemist) that could even come close to duplicating what the mother's body produces.

The two exercises that I recommend to my patients are walking or swimming simply because they are both low impact on the body. Walking in water is wonderful if you are having pain in your lower legs or back because the buoyancy of the water keeps much of the weight off your feet and legs. You just get into water at about chest level and walk. This is just as good for you as walking on the ground because you are now pushing against the water that compensates for the buoyancy. With walking you don't even need anything special except good shoes. I know we are accustomed to having a "sports uniform" for each exercise but walking does not require any of that.

It does not matter how fast you walk either because the physical benefit is measured by distance times mass (weight). I know it seems that you are doing more if you run, but the only benefit is that you can run the distance faster than you can walk it. My patients often say but you sweat when you run. Actually, you also sweat (perspire) when you walk but it is slow enough that it evaporates before becoming noticeable like it does when you run. If it is cold you just layer up for walking. I prefer just casual clothing with a zip-up hoodie. You start with the hood up and then as your warm up you just take the hood down which allows a great deal of body heat to escape (something like 25-30%). As you get even warmer you just unzip the hoodie to allow your abdominal body heat to escape more readily then as you get even warmer you remove the hoodie. This simple layering helps with the "logistics" of the equipment.

Push your body

One way to increase your exercise routine is to look for ways to exercise anytime you can, even at work. Take the stairs as often as possible or if you have the opportunity to carry something rather than using a cart then take the "difficult way out" for yourself. Walking at lunch or on a break is far better than just sitting still during that time. It can shorten the time you need to exercise before or after work. Exercise is cumulative in that is almost as useful to exercise for several times a day as it is to exercise for longer one time a day. Again walking is a good opportunity to exercise during the day without having to change into your workout clothes. If your work is somewhat physical then do all of it that you can and think of it as getting paid while you work rather than having to pay a fee to join a health facility. So the bottom line here is don't even look for the easy way to do something if it is physical but seek avenues that can allow you some physical challenge.

Nutrition/Diet

Our bodies are wonderful "machines" of high complexity that works so very well when we take good care of them. But, often we do not appreciate the basic needs of the workings of the body and attempt to take shortcuts to achieve our physical goals. The body's needs are rather simple but we fill them with so much "junk" that it is amazing that they function at all. The body has an amazing capacity to compensate for other parts of the body that may be struggling but it can only perform "extra duty" for so many years, and then it seems that everything begins to fail at once...which is essentially true.

It would be best for our body's health and maximum efficiency if we only put food and water into it, if possible. I recognize so very well that there are some needs for the body to have medicines to function well but there are even many of those ailments that might have been avoided if we taken better care of our bodies in the past. A prime example of damage to the body is whenever a person is diagnosed with high blood pressure and does not take their medicines. We do not know what causes most cases of high blood pressure because even young athletes can have it, but if you do know that you have this dangerous condition it is imperative that you keep it under control. With hypertension you don't feel anything until the levels become very high and enough to feel dizzy or a headache and that is often just prior to a stroke. That is why hypertension is called the "silent killer" and it deserves this name.

The way I attempt to relate to patients about one of the biggest dangers of hypertension is the damage it does to the kidneys. I usually hold up a sheet of paper and show them that blood flows by one side and urine is on the other with the paper serving as a filter to allow the waste products from the blood to pass through the filter and be excreted in the urine. Then I demonstrate that if the blood flow (high blood pressure) "beats up" this very fine and fragile filter for so long the body goes into kidney failure. One day you are feeling well and the next you are looking at kidney dialysis or a kidney transplant because the untreated hypertension destroyed all those wonderful filters. I also tell them you can have "flame hemorrhages" in the interior of the eye and that is why providers look into the eyeball to observe any damage to the eye tissue. Of course there is also the damage to your heart and complete circulatory system because there is too much pressure on the entire system.

One of the very best ways to reduce hypertension is to get your stress under control the very best that you can and exercise as well as lose weight, if necessary. There have been follow-up studies to show that we don't need to worry about the salt content as much as we previously believed. It is possible to learn to use less salt on or in your food but it is not as much of a contributor to hypertension as earlier believed.

Unfortunately, every medicine has at least one side effect and most medicines are almost "scary" when you read all the things that could go wrong if you take the prescribed medicines. That is why an excellent goal for you and yours is to take no medicines or to attempt to take the very least of any medicine that you can to achieve the desired result. I have had many patients come to me with a bag of prescription bottles and many of them they don't even know what they are for. When I took many of them away that needed to be eliminated they were very thankful and would tell me on their next visit that they often now felt better. I am very blessed that I don't take any medicines on a routine basis. I do take antihistamines during the spring and fall seasons if needed. I know that many people have problems that require medicines in order to survive, but there are so many things we can do to preserve the natural integrity of the body that can keep us from having to put another foreign substance into this wonderful machine. I wish everyone could take an anatomy and physiology class to understand what amazing systems we have and how they work together, because the better you understand the body, the more you will want to protect it from outside influences (like undue stress) and foreign substances.

As a part of our medical training, we had to take a course in nutrition. That was an excellent course because you study the different systems that have to do with nutrition as well as what certain foods do to the body. It was interesting to learn that you can obtain every nutrient that the body needs to sustain life from rice and beans. You might tire of the lack of change of diet, but you could still live and on just those two foods. It is also interesting that both of those foods are very inexpensive and easy to transport when dried. This allows us to provide adequate food for much of the poorer part of the world more easily and economically. It was also enlightening that broccoli was the leader in several different categories of beneficial foods. You are also exposed to the glycemic quotient of food that helps explain why you need to eat again soon after eating rice.

If you eat properly, you do not need any vitamin or supplement unless you are diagnosed with some type of deficiency. I know that many medical people tout vitamins and supplements, especially if they have a financial interest in you using them, but there have not been any well-documented experiments or well-controlled studies to indicate that vitamins have made a nutritional difference. Those who sell them will tell you differently, of course, and will attempt to convince you that I am giving you bad advice. They may tell you about a person who now feels so much better after taking

NUTRITION/DIET

the vitamin or supplement, but many of these supplements do not contain what they claim and often do not have the level advertised. Often, they use an anecdotal example of how Grandpa is now feeling so much better since he started taking this new miracle drug. Well, in truth, Grandpa may have a new *girlfriend* who is making him feel so much better, and that is why any study needs hundreds of patients to provide a good study.

I have some personal experience with vitamins. On two different occasions (several years apart), I was told that if I tried these vitamins for thirty days, they would guarantee that I would feel better or they would give me my money back, which I think is a wonderful idea and that is why this book has a money-back guarantee. After taking the different brand vitamins for the full thirty-day period, I did not feel any better nor did I feel any worse when I stopped. Another longer term experiment was for six years. While I was in medical training, I was informed about a global study for prostate cancer. I have never had a problem with that, and I knew that all studies need as many well patients as they do ill patients, so I joined the study. We had to take vitamins every morning, but we did not know if this general vitamin contained either vitamin E or selenium. The study was stopped after I was in it for six (long) years because they found that the study was causing problems! I did not feel better when I started taking the vitamins, and I did not feel worse when I stopped taking them after six years. My personal experience matters little to an academic-approved study, but neither my personal experience nor controlled studies demonstrate any real benefit to the vitamin or supplement plans.

Also, be aware that the actual active ingredient in a pill is a very small part of the bulk of the pill and most of it is filler. So, once again you are putting a foreign substance into your body. I again ask you to consider making your body a "drug-free zone" if possible. If it is necessary that you take medicine, then take the very least dose you can to achieve the desired results. Some providers seem to give a pill for everything rather than take the time to discuss life changes because it takes more time, and most patients don't follow the advice anyway.

Water

Water is one of the most important items we can discuss in our efforts to reduce stress! Experts tell us that our bodies are somewhere around 70-75% water, so therefore water warrants our attention. Even our bones are mostly water, and certainly the rest of our body is more obviously water-filled.

I conducted a year-long study of water consumption of over 400 of my patients. We performed a urinalysis on every patient at mostly my expense if their insurance did not cover it. I selected specific gravity for an appropriate measure of water consumption. Specific gravity is a measure of how dense (non-diluted) the urine is. I chose to use a specific gravity of 1.030 or higher as "dehydrated." Two-thirds (67% or two out of three) of my patients measured 1.030 or higher (which was higher than the instrument could measure)! If we moved down one notch to 1.025 as a reading, 75% (three out of four) were inadequately hydrated!

I waited a few months and repeated the test again with a total testing time of one year. During that year we tested every patient (mostly at my expense) for adequate hydration. The last month-long test of over 400 patients had reduced the inadequately hydrated group to fewer than 15%. This was partially due to my "hounding" the patients to drink more water. I was amazed how many patients told me that they *never* drink water! But they would bring their opened bottle of a caffeinated, carbonated, warm drink with them to the visit.

I had one twenty-year-old female who had passed a total of

eleven kidney stones already! She was "off the chart" and over the capacity of the instrument to even read, so I was not able to tell her how high she was, but it was certainly *too* high. I discussed her water consumption (or lack of) and explained all the damage that could be done to her kidneys by inadequate hydration. Her next visit she was again off the chart, so I had another long discussion with her and pointed out that when a kidney stone is forming, it is also damaging kidney tissue. Her third visit she was again off the chart. I was appalled! To finally get her attention, I told her that if she came back that dehydrated again, I would dismiss her as a patient. Now *she* was appalled, but I explained that I would do the same if she were supposed to take blood pressure medicine and did not for three straight visits. This time she took my advice and was never that dehydrated again, nor did she have a kidney stone after focusing on drinking more water.

Why don't healthcare providers talk about water consumption more? It is not because they don't realize the value of proper hydration, but there is such a low success rate of having patients comply, and it takes too long to discuss this very simple health need.

You can't make much progress here unless the patient gets on board because some patients have not drunk water by itself in years. Water is so very important to so many of our body systems. Often when a patient complained of constipation, I would ask how much water they drank, and the answer was nearly always disappointing to me. When food is in the stomach, it is mostly water. When the food moves into the small intestine, it is still mostly water. When it leaves the small intestine to move into the large intestine, it is still mostly water. In the large intestine the body starts withdrawing the water to reuse for other systems. All of this is normal, and when you are adequately hydrated, the large intestine does not remove any more water than is necessary because the brain is telling it to do so and your fecal material is not hard and formed.

When you are constipated the first suspect should be inadequate hydration. If now you take a stimulant laxative, you are causing even more trauma to your body because you are causing it to react to a stimulant medicine rather than a natural process with adequate hydration. There are other things that cause constipation, like other medications, which is another reason to minimize taking any drugs you safely can. If you are taking medications that have a side effect of constipation, then you need to increase your water consumption even more.

How can you tell you are adequately hydrated without running a test on your urine? It is so simple to get an excellent reading of your level of hydration if you will just observe your urine (easier for males of course). If it is almost clear, then you are more than likely well hydrated. If it is dark or yellow (except the morning void when you have not been drinking water during the night), you need to drink probably two to three times the water you currently are, until your urine becomes almost clear. **How simple is that?** But yet many people do not realize the value of being adequately hydrated and are not willing to drink enough water. Their excuse is that they drink other fluids, and that is important, but many other drinks, while being mostly water, have chemicals in them that cause the body to urinate even more to attempt to eliminate the chemicals.

It is possible to be overhydrated (water intoxication, water poisoning, or dilutional hyponatremia). This is a danger because it causes the body to lose important and essential electrolytes that are necessary for the body organs to function. I have only seen one case of this situation, and it was a patient I saw in the emergency room due to this problem. His urine was totally clear! His family members accompanied him to the ER and related that this was a problem for him for years and that he would drink water directly out of the toilet tank if they did not give him water. He had been in therapy and institutionalized more than once for this problem due to the medical danger of electrolyte deficiency. I never had a patient in any of my clinics with this problem, so it is a very rare problem and not one to use as an excuse for adequate hydration.

When we breathe out, we lose water. That is why you can cloud up your glasses to assist in cleaning them or to write on a glass. All night long your body loses water in this fashion as well as evaporation. So when you awaken in the morning, your urine should be the densest of any time of the day and therefore darker. Your body craves water! It has functioned for hours without any additional water, so certainly it is recycling water from your large intestine. Often we go to bed without having adequately hydrated for several hours because we don't want to have to awaken to urinate.

It is critical that your body gets water the first thing in the morning! But often the water it does receive is laced with caffeine or other stimulants like sugar because it gives you that quick (but empty) energy. If you are thirsty, that is a sure sign you are already well on your way to dehydration, so it is time to find the nearest water bottle and drink it. I am also amazed when I ask patients about their water consumption and they tell me how many bottles they have in their refrigerator or in their car, but when I ask them how many of these bottles they consume, they are not really drinking any more than before. Unfortunately, the only way you can get water into your system is to drink it unless you have an IV (intravenous) intervention to overcome your dehydration. When I worked in the ER, it was eye-opening to the patients (and providers) what a difference they felt after a bag or two of saline had dripped into their veins!

I keep a gallon of water on my bathroom counter at room temperature. It is easier to drink more water if it is at room temperature because the coldness of the water does not cause pain to the throat. I recognize this may sound gross to you, but I drink straight from the gallon jug...sorry about that revelation that you did not care to know. I turn the jug up and chug-a-lug for several seconds and consume well over 20 ounces quickly. There is an almost immediate "cascade of coolness" that I feel after giving my body the very item it needs most upon awakening. I have read of others who have experienced the same cool feeling when they hydrate early after awakening, so it is not a sensation that only I feel. I challenge you to attempt something similar. You may prefer to have a small bottle of water rather than a jug, but the main goal is to consume a good portion of water upon awakening. The body will quickly process it out of your stomach so it will not interfere with your breakfast. In just a few days of this new hydration routine, the benefit will become more obvious and hopefully you will feel the cascade of coolness also.

On two different occasions I have been selected to do a random urinary drug screen and my urine sample had been too dilute! So, all I had to do was wait a few hours until my urine could concentrate more and I passed without any problem. This was due to my early morning cascade of coolness and testing early in the morning. I don't plan to change my morning water chugging because of the good benefits, but if I am chosen for random drug testing again, I will just test later in the day.

I have a condition called hypoglycemia, which is where it seems your body makes too much insulin, and when I take in too much sugar (or much of any sugar), the output from the pancreas is too great for the sugar load. The excess insulin burns the sugar up so rapidly that I go into a "low sugar" state similar to diabetes. Many medical providers don't quite understand hypoglycemia (low blood sugar) and often respond by saying, "We will just give you some candy or sugar-loaded food so your blood glucose (sugar) load will come up." And it will temporarily, but then I will produce too much insulin and will fall to an even lower sugar level! One of the complications to hypoglycemia is that later you can develop hyperglycemia (diabetes). Then your medical life really becomes complicated!

One of the symptoms of diabetes is continual thirst, and this is used to assist in making the diagnosis of diabetes along with some other laboratory tests.

Several years ago I noticed that I was drinking more water but still feeling thirsty. Fortunately, one of our national meetings that year was in California, and DuPont hired some experts to speak to us about our overall health. This expense and time was again justified by the thought that if you are healthy and feel good, you can be a better, more productive employee. One of the speakers focused on water consumption but also stressed using distilled water. Distilled water is water that has been heated enough to become steam and then subjected to a cold object that causes the steam (vapor) to condense again to a liquid. This process is used in many areas of chemistry to "purify" a combination of chemicals. You can distill the filthiest water you can find, but the water that condenses back to liquid will always be pure water with no ions (electrolytes) in it.

My first thought was "I bet that distilled water tastes terrible!" I was mistaken! It is as tasteful as other water, at least to me. Often water's taste is determined by the contaminants found there or even put there purposefully by the manufacturer. I remember several years ago when they found out a very expensive water (Perrier) had a unique taste because it contained low levels of benzene, which is a hydrocarbon that is very harmful to the body. The interesting thing to me about drinking distilled water was that I demonstrated to myself that the feeling of being thirsty all the time went away just as the speaker had said when I started drinking the distilled water!

If you have ever allowed a drop of tap water or even any water other than distilled water to evaporate on a stainless steel or dark-colored surface, you will notice a white residue that is often difficult to remove once it is dried. Well, if greater than 70% of our bodies is water, I want the purest, cleanest water available to make up that high percentage! If there is that much residue from just a few drops, how much is there in 20 ounces of water that your body has to process and eliminate if not needed? So I switched to distilled water immediately and drink it most of the time. I drink other water when at restaurants or when I am not at home near my gallon container, but I cannot tell the difference in the taste. Others say that they can, and even so, I ask you to make a concerted effort to switch to distilled water most of the time so that nothing but the purest water goes into your body.

I have had patients and seminar participants say that they are worried about not getting the fluoride needed for strong teeth if they switch to distilled water. You will get less fluoride, but you will still get an adequate amount for that protection from the other water and other drinks that are mostly water. Just look at the label on any water you consume (and I want you to consider consuming more, if needed) and see what the ingredients are. On distilled water the only ingredient is water! All other waters that are labeled have to list the other ingredients, and most often we don't need them in our wonderful bodies. Distilled water is usually the same price as other water, which is amazing to me since it requires a heating and cooling process that other waters do not. A gallon is often less than a dollar at discount stores. When I buy my distilled water, it is often almost a shopping cart full. People often question me about why I am buying so much, and I usually say that I do a lot of ironing to get them to smile because few people on the planet iron anymore and most of them are women. Then I tell them the benefits of the distilled water. The reason you should use distilled water in any appliance that causes evaporation is that the waste products (scale) will stop up your iron and sometimes cause problems with other appliances. So, again, if the scale from the water stops up appliances, why should my body process that same waste product? And why process so much of it? It was an easy choice for me and I hope it is for you also.

There are many benefits to drinking enough water and if you want to know all or more of them, just search the Web. You will find far more there than I plan to discuss here, but I do want to ask you to take my suggestion to heart and just go ahead and drink, drink, drink more water. Most people and patients I have talked to about water consumption need to drink three times as much as they currently consume. You need to learn to "chug" the water instead of just sipping it because the sipping technique will consume too much time and not deliver enough water to your body. My twelve-year-old granddaughter has had a problem with drinking water for most of her life and did experience several kidney infections when younger that could have been attributed to inadequate hydration. Now we have a rule that she has to drink at least a 20-ounce bottle of water before she gets out of the car for school.

Another visible sign of inadequate hydration is if someone has "wrinkled" lips. This is not an absolute, but it works most of the time. When your brain needs water to function, it will extract it from other parts of the body so it can function properly, and the lips are often a visible sign. So, even if it is not definite proof, then at least consider it a warning sign. Seldom do we drink too much water, if ever.

A book entitled *Your Body's Many Cries for Water*, written by Fereydoon Batmanghelidj, MD, has some good suggestions about water consumption. He was a prisoner in Iran and was told to help the other prisoners with their health problems. He had no medicines so he began to focus on the benefits of water consumption. Many of his fellow prisoners were complaining of stomach problems. He started having them drink a great deal of water, and most of their abdominal complaints subsided. That is a reasonable conclusion because the stomach acid can become very concentrated if the brain has the body pull the water out of that reservoir of liquid, thereby making the liquid stored there more acidic. When you drink more water quickly, you automatically dilute the stomach acid and cause the acidity to drop and become less of a problem. I have demonstrated this on myself many times, even with the emphasis I put on adequate hydration. I find that consuming a goodly amount of water does most often help the few times I experience an upset stomach.

The author of this book has many good suggestions about the benefits of drinking water that I have confirmed personally and in research with my patients, but some of the other data he espouses is not supported adequately by research. So, I don't agree with everything he states, but he does have several excellent points.

As people age, they lose some of their ability to sense thirst and forget to hydrate adequately. If you have any influence with an older person (even if it is yourself), then please encourage adequate hydration. Water is an excellent insulator and helps retain body heat, so if an older person is having difficulty staying warm, they might benefit from more water consumption. That is such an amazing fix! Water is cheaper than any other drink and does so very much for us that hopefully we will do better about drinking *just* water. This is a decision that helps me feel so confident in giving a money-back guarantee to you because so few people are aware of the need or benefits of adequate hydration.

What about "vitamin water" or sugar-laced drinks? You just have to consider what the additives are doing for you, or to you. I don't recommend vitamins in any form except natural food, so I see no benefit of drinking a vitamin dissolved in water. The sugar and flavoring and even the coloring in other drinks are just something else your wonderful body has to deal with. Our bodies already have to deal with so much; why should we make it more difficult for such an amazing "factory" that keeps us going all day?

Allergies are certainly reduced with more hydration! I know this and have proven it to myself over and over. When my ears feel as if they are stopping up, I go for the water and start chugging. This has two benefits. The first is that the water thins the mucous membranes that go throughout the body so the mucous is more easily disposed of by the body. The second is that the swallowing mechanism helps equate the feeling of increased pressure in the middle ear just like swallowing does when you are changing altitude. If you have ever experienced these symptoms you will be amazed with the change if you start chugging water. I have timed the results, and it has never been more than 20 minutes before I feel some relief, and most often at ten to fifteen minutes. In addition, if you are adequately hydrated, the mucous membranes of the nasal passages are more liquid, so when an allergen comes into contact with the mucous membrane, it can be "flushed out" and down into the stomach to be excreted. This happens before allergens can "bore through" the mucous membrane to get into the bloodstream and cause a histamine reaction that you now have to take an antihistamine medicine to overcome. You might be able to avoid antihistamines totally if you can be proactive and stay adequately hydrated during the pollen season. I drink even more water in the spring and fall just to minimize the allergic reaction that is so very uncomfortable and actually is often just a miserable time of the season.

When I was in high school, the allergies would totally zap my energy and make me miserable with itchy eyes. I would sit down to study and nothing would go into my brain. I was a fair student in high school and had a reasonably easy time with even my science and math classes, but my grades would have greatly improved if I had been able to avoid or treat my springtime allergies. I would go into the final with a good grade but would do poorly on the spring final and most often would drop a letter grade for the semester based on the final test. I would spend time studying for the spring exams just like I would for the fall final exams, but I was not able to absorb the content that normally came to me easily enough to allow me to enjoy school without killing myself with studying. Actually, I would study more in the spring but would still not do as well on the final. On top of that I would find that if I had made an "A" in a course the first half of the year but would most often drop to a "B" the second half and then I would receive a "B" for the entire year! I asked my guidance counselor about this situation and she said the school policy was that if you made a higher grade the last half of the year, you would get the higher grade for the entire year. But if you made a lower grade the last half of the year than you did the first, they averaged it to the lower grade because it demonstrated you were not doing as well and were not making progress; whereas if you made a higher grade the second half than you did the first, you were showing improvement! So my allergies at the very end of the school year were lowering my overall grade for the entire year! I experienced the same difficulty studying on the final for college, but there the spring semester was not "averaged" with the first or fall semester.

If you or your children are struggling at times, especially in the spring or fall, I would greatly encourage you to get tested for allergies. You may not realize how badly you feel until you start feeling so much better!

I want to re-emphasis that you should "protect" your body to preserve its natural state as much as possible. This effort is tantamount to you reducing stress because if your body is stressed physically and emotionally, you will suffer greatly as you are attempting to do better. Even worse is if you become ill due to this "abuse" of your body; then you have to deal with your previous stress and you have the added burden of the stress-induced medical problem. Please think of what you are putting into your body each and every time you put anything there that your body has to deal with. Every medicine, whether a prescription, over-the-counter, or herbal, may have some negative effect on the body to cancel some of the positive benefits. Also remember that any controlled substance must have some danger or it would not be controlled by the governing bodies.

Often patients do not realize what medicines do to their body to achieve the desired results. I tell them that when they take any level of opiate to help with pain, the medicine is not reducing the pain or the cause of the pain, but is only altering their brain to make it think it is not feeling pain. Pain is very useful to tell us something is wrong. Actually, when you are examining a patient and they say that this movement is causing pain, then at least it means that the nerves are working, which is very important because if they are not "firing," the muscles and bones are not going to move. You need to determine what is causing the pain and do anything you can to reduce or minimize it. Even adequate hydration can help here if you are experiencing back pain because the water can more adequately "swell" the disks between the vertebrae. Often pain is due to, or certainly made worse by, undue stress, so reducing stress can lessen pain. And reducing pain can reduce stress, so if something as simple as more water can help reduce your back pain, then your stress can also diminish.

Eliminate or reduce anything you possibly can to help restore the body to a more natural level of balance. I am not touting some special routine or medicine. I am simply asking you to put only proper food and the purest water you can into your body. This is such a basic "truth" that is overlooked in our busy, over media-saturated lives where we are bombarded with taking this or that supplement or drinking a beverage to make us feel better when the consequences of doing so far outweigh the benefits.

Reduce

If you really want to reduce your stress level, you need to begin with the basic question of "**WHY**" do you do anything in your life that does not reduce your stress. We will discuss several topics that can best be understood if we answer the basic question of "why do I need or desire this." You will be amazed how this opens your mind to suggestions to change when you examine this fundamental question of "why?"

Alcohol

To have a healthier, longer, less stressed life, you need to ask yourself the fundamental question, "Why do I even need alcohol?" This is a critical, crucial question to ask that can affect your life and the lives around you! Why do *you* need it? If you can't answer the question quickly, then I implore you, for your sake, to spend the time determining the answer to that important question. This question can change your life for the positive in so many ways that you won't understand until you make this life-changing move.

Alcoholism was so prevalent in my mother's side of the family that it ruined several of her brothers' lives. Her oldest brother was dismissed from the Army at nineteen years and nine months, thereby keeping him from gaining retirement. He must have really messed up to be discharged that close to retirement because it is my understanding that years ago, as well as now, the military "take care of their own." He later in life would drink anything that had any level of alcohol, including hair tonic, if he could not get to beer or whisky. My mother had eight brothers, and all of them drank a great deal of alcohol. Three were able to stop and went on to become very successful businessmen even without a formal education. The other five ruined their lives and often their families' lives also by excessive drinking. My mother told me all about this when I was a youngster, and I made the decision that if they could not handle alcohol, then I was not any better or stronger than they were, so I would not be able to do any better than the worst of them. I honestly believe that even now with all the supposed maturity I should have, if I started drinking I would become addicted. Many older retired people who did not have a problem with alcohol in their earlier years have a real problem later because they have more time and money to be able to drink more without others knowing about it.

I have never tasted beer and only whisky when my father mixed "rock candy" in it as a cough suppressant. Even that small amount made me very sleepy. I have had a few sips of wine simply due to my entertaining in the corporate world since it is such a social part of the meal. I am not "Mr. Goody-Two Shoes" here because I have certainly made other serious mistakes in my life, but I have never regretted the decision not to drink.

Alcohol is a depressant!!!! So rather than making you feel better, it depresses your senses and makes you think you are doing well. It is impossible to reason with someone who has a drinking problem. When they are under the influence, they can't understand anything you are saying to get them to understand the problem they are causing, and when they are sober, they can't understand why you are upset at them because they don't remember anything they did when under the influence. A famous actor only believed his children's stories of his drunken actions after they videotaped him to show him when he was sober what a changed person he was when he was drunk.

We all know truly tragic stories of how alcohol "mistakes" have caused ruin to so many others. Just recently I treated a female patient for anxiety due to a young man, under the influence, killing her husband, a young woman he had helped with her car problems, and her unborn child. The driver left the scene, so he is charged with that and three counts of vehicular homicide as well as millions of dollars in lawsuits against him and his family, who had the vehicle in their name. So aside from the terrible, tragic deaths of the three people he killed due to drinking, he now has very serious criminal charges against him. His family will never recover from the lawsuits, so everything they ever gained is now lost, as well as the freedom of their child, who is now a young adult! I know you probably know of more devastating stories than these, so please tell yourself that you have the potential for doing the same thing at some time in the future.

You can sometimes tell if someone drives under the influence often, even if they are never caught or cause a major problem, because their car usually has small, minor dents all over it where they have misjudged the distance to another object while drinking. One night I followed a man for over 40 minutes through two counties weaving all over the road and nearly having an accident with every car he met. Because he changed counties and was on rural roads, he was able to pull into his driveway before the local law enforcement officers caught him. They talked to him but could not arrest him because they had not observed him themselves and could not take my word for his endangering so many others that night.

Alcohol has a chemical structure of an –OH group or one oxygen and one hydrogen atom attached to a carbon chain that has two carbons in it. So it is essentially two carbons, an –OH group and several hydrogen atoms attached. This is called ethyl alcohol, signifying a two-carbon chain with an –OH group attached. If you only have one carbon with an –OH group, you have methyl alcohol, which will cause blindness if you drink it. If the carbon chain has three carbons either in a straight line (n-propyl) or forked chain (isopropyl or rubbing alcohol), you will die if you drink enough. This recently happened to numerous people in India and can happen to anyone who purchases illegal alcohol. So you have a liquid that will make you go blind if it has one carbon, a depressant that can cause alcoholic poisoning in excess if it has two carbons, and death if it has three carbons attached to the –OH group then the entire group is bad for you. Some organic chemistry books relate that ethyl alcohol is the least poisonous of all the liquid alcohols. What is consumed as alcohol may be the least poisonous, but it is still poisonous! So you are putting a known poison into your body each and every time you drink alcohol. It is so sad to see patients with greatly enlarged livers because their liver is damaged so much that it has to become larger to function properly.

The next step of damage to the liver is called cirrhosis, and if severe enough it will so damage the liver tissue that the liver cannot process <u>any</u> of the drugs you may need for your heart, high blood pressure, diabetes, pain or any prescribed medicine because all of these are "broken down" in the liver to give your body their benefit. If you need alcohol to help you unwind or face the day, then again you need to ask the question "why do I need this?" There are other ways to unwind and face the day, and we will discuss them here. They are so very simplistic in their implementation but have such wonderful results.

Alcohol addiction or overuse can best be controlled by attending Alcoholic Anonymous meetings regularly. This is the most successful process that has been developed, and you may need to attend a meeting a day for the rest of your life, if necessary, to control this problem. It is a small price to pay for the difficulties that alcohol can cause. I love one of this successful program's phrases, "One drink is too many and a thousand is not enough!" This is so true for many other problems we face in our lives.

Nicotine (Smoking Is Soooooooooo Stupid!)

I do so dislike the word "stupid." It ranks right up there with "ugly." Neither of these words needs to be in our vocabulary because of the negative connotation associated with them, but honestly, smoking deserves the use of this word. Here is another place that you need to ask yourself "Why?" This is the most addictive drug available without a prescription, in my opinion. I have formed this stance based on what hundreds of my patients have told me, not on my own research. In spite of the other times in my life where I was "an abject fool," I have never smoked and I am glad on a daily basis for this when I see the struggle of very strong people attempting to overcome this addiction. I have had hundreds of patients tell me that they stopped alcohol or illegal drugs but could not stop smoking, and I can believe that. I have had three patients tell me that they were able to stop using "crack" cocaine (one had even been a dealer) but could not stop smoking.

If you want a better understanding of why nicotine is so addictive, get the movie *The Insider* with Russell Crowe and Al Pacino starring in the major roles. Crowe's character is a chemist in the tobacco industry who learns that they are putting ammonia compounds into the tobacco to allow the nicotine to more readily cross the blood-brain barrier, thereby increasing the strength of the addiction. Also it has lately been revealed that tobacco now has more nicotine than previously.

I had one of my staff look at the patients listed in my practice of the medically underserved (who are also usually of lower economic means) who smoke divided by the total number of patients, which would allow me to calculate the percentage of smokers in my total practice. The results were absolutely astounding! I knew the numbers would be high because I discussed this so often with my patients, and it seemed that at times I was discussing this with almost every patient. The results of the survey showed that 88% of my patients smoked! That is over four times the national average of approximately 20% and well over three times the Tennessee state average of approximately 25%! I spent many cumulative hours discussing ways to stop this addiction but with limited success. Some patients even told me that they had no intention of stopping due to the good feeling nicotine gave them.

The U.S. government used to give cigarettes to soldiers, and I have seen the government-issued packs in a museum in Anchorage, Alaska. I have heard the stories of older military veterans who started smoking while in the military because you were able to take longer breaks if it was a "smoke break." Cigarettes were so inexpensive, anyone could afford all they wanted. Japan used to encourage smoking because the workers who smoked were more productive. I wonder what the Japanese and U.S. military think of that decision now that they have to take care of the medical needs of those long-term smokers.

I conducted research on 150 smoking patients in an industrial plant to see the success rate of smoking cessation using Chantix,® a drug that blocks the receptors in the brain where the nicotine attaches. My results verified what the manufacturer claimed, so the research was considered successful. The plant paid for the drug (all except $3.00 per month) to help the employees stop smoking. As a part of my counseling with some of them, I looked into the cost saving with them. One couple was spending over $600 per month (these are after-tax dollars so their real cost would be a good deal more). They were amazed at their expense. This was a motivator for them to stop as well as all the other benefits that we will not discuss here.

Most smokers know the damage of smoking and the benefits of stopping but still can't seem to quit. I often ask the smoking patients if I built a fire in the office and fed tobacco leaves to keep it going, would they stay in the office with me? The answer is always a resounding NO! Then I point out that smoking is even worse because they are drawing this smoke directly into their lungs as opposed to inhaling it from the open fire, which is essentially secondhand smoke.

Then I ask them how you get a cigarette going or started. They tell me that they use a match or lighter. I become as dramatic as I can and say, "So you are telling me that you have to set this tobacco (and paper) on FIRE! Now you are inhaling the combustion gases of a FIRE down into your lungs, and if you don't inhale deeply, it will go out and you have to apply more FIRE to restart the process!" They seem so surprised when I reduce the process to that level of simplicity.

How do you stop smoking? First, ask yourself the basic questions—why did you start and why do you keep smoking when almost everyone knows the dangers of doing so? After you identify the answers, you have to have a TOTAL commitment to quit completely. No process, even with the success of the prescription drugs to assist in this process, works unless you are fully committed to stopping. I do hope you are successful, and if you are, you can tell yourself that you are one of the strongest-willed people on this entire planet because so few are able to stop smoking even when they have been successful stopping other addictions.

Research has shown that there are no known cases of anyone smoking marijuana who did not start with smoking cigarettes first. This is an excellent reason to keep our young people from starting smoking because it can also help deal with another addictive problem.

I really hate to write these next few lines because I love people so much that it is not good for me! Smokers, you stink! Your hair stinks, your breath stinks, your skin stinks, your clothes stink, your homes and cars stink! Cigarette smoke even stinks outside if you have to walk near it. As a provider, as I am listening to the patient's breath sounds it requires that my face is somewhat close to their hair when I have my stethoscope on their back. If they are a smoker and especially if they haven't washed their hair recently, the odor almost makes me ill. Of course they can't smell the odor because their smelling sensation is reduced by their smoking. I always keep a can of air freshener to use after a smoker leaves my office, and I get to use it often, unfortunately.

Smokers don't realize that they have lost the ability to smell normally that may be due to the vasoconstrictive properties of the nicotine. That is why previous smokers often comment that food taste better after they stop smoking. Much of the taste of food is due to the odor that the food has so if a smoker's sense of smell is reduced by the nicotine then food will taste better after cessation of smoking.

One of the worst for women smokers is the damage it does to the skin on their face by causing wrinkles. I call it the "smoker's mask" where when they smile you can see the muscles under the skin move, but the wrinkled skin does not. This just kills me, for so many lovely women (whom society judges so very much on their looks) now look much older than their age. The skin even changes color due to smoking. When a person stops smoking, you will soon see the difference in skin color, and it usually starts in the cheeks. It is as if they are wearing blush, when in reality the blood is no longer carrying the poisons around to feed the skin.

With male smokers I often ask if they know what Viagra® is,

and the usual response is, "I don't need that stuff!" I then explain how smoking is a vasoconstrictor (which means the blood flow is reduced) and that could reduce the blood flow to a very important part of their anatomy as well as a reduced blood flow to the sphincter muscle that traps the blood in the penis, allowing an erection. I don't really know of any definitive proof of this, but it seems a reasonable thought since we know that blood flow is reduced with smokers so much that some surgeries, especially the hands, often will not be performed on smokers. This is due to the lack of blood flow to the extremities so the healing process will not be successful. This may seem to be a scare tactic to stop men from smoking, but it does succeed in having them think about the consequences of nicotine consumption as it does for women to realize that their looks will be impacted negatively.

Reynaud's disease leads to a reduction of blood flow to the hands and fingers, causing the extremities to appear blue and cold. This is a very painful condition. Some drugs can cause this, but often it is due to the vasoconstrictive properties of the nicotine. I have had several patients with this painful disease who are still smokers!

Capillary Refill

One of my favorite ways of physically demonstrating the problems with smoking and adequate blood flow is called "capillary refill." Have you wondered why the hospital requires that a surgical patient remove their nail polish prior to surgery? A trained medical person can tell how well your body is receiving adequate blood and oxygen flow by looking at your nails. If they are nice and pink, then your blood flow there, as well as the rest of your body, is adequate. If your nails are bluish and not a healthy pink, they know immediately that there is a problem with your circulation and/or oxygenation.

Have you ever noticed that when you squeeze your fingernail, it turns white and then returns to pink after you release the pressure? When you put pressure on your nail, you squeeze the blood out of the capillaries and cause them to become white. "Capillary refill" is a measure of how long it takes for your nails to turn pink after pressure is released. A smoker's capillary refill time will usually be longer than a non-smoker's. I use this method to indicate to smokers how my capillary refill is much faster even if I am a few decades older than they are. A non-smoker's capillary refill is almost instantaneous, whereas a smoker's will take longer. This is a very powerful way of demonstrating how much nicotine is causing a reduction in the blood flow to your body, but is most evident in the extremities. Long-term smokers may actually have white fingernail beds to alert providers that this person has circulatory problems. There are other factors that compromise your capillary refill, but even those indicate there is a problem with your circulation.

I also ask those who have poor capillary refill time where else in the body that the poor circulation could impact, and few of them answer the entire circulatory system. This effect is also easily seen when the medical provider looks into the eyeball to see the overall health of your entire circulatory system.

Clubbing

This is not a suggestion for something to do for entertainment. This is a very sad effect of poor circulation for whatever reason, but it is most often caused by nicotine's vasoconstrictive impact on blood flow to the fingers. Clubbing is where the last digit of your finger is now larger than it used to be and can be significantly bigger than the other digits of your fingers. The ends of the nail begin to curve downward, and the entire nail begins to become more curved also. Look this up on the Internet if you want an example of what this looks like. The very worst part about this is that even if you stop smoking, your fingers will not return to their normal state but will retain this "clubbing" forever. I have had some patients become so very aware of the look of their fingers that it is a major motivator for them to stop even further damage, but it is also a sad reminder of what they have done to their body—you cannot hide your hands from others like you can some other physical manifestation.

YouTube Demo

One reason I never smoked was because when I was fourteen years old, I started working at a full-service gasoline station where we did the car washes by hand. There was always a film that was hard to remove from the windows of the smokers' cars. It took a great deal more time to remove this film because it was tar-like and not the usual dirt on the glass, so you had to use stronger chemicals to remove it. I decided then (since I was having to work harder to remove this film) to never smoke because if it was on the glass, then what would it do to my lungs?

On YouTube there is an excellent demo of the junk that is in the lungs after just one cigarette. There are two two-liter bottles filled with water and connected by clear tubing that comes together in a Y shape. A cigarette is placed in one single tube of the y-tubing. The bottoms of the two bottles are now pierced to allow the water to drain out and actually smoke the cigarette that is now lit. When the water drains out of the two bottles, they are full of smoke. The junction of the y-tube now has visible residue. The researchers remove the tops from each of the bottles and force the smoke through a white cloth, which demonstrates ugly brown residue from just one cigarette! This is a very powerful demonstration, and I encourage everyone to look at it even if you are a non-smoker.

I remember when you could smoke in an airplane, and I was forced to be exposed to all that recirculating contamination. My hands were always dirty after the flight when I washed them. Since my hands are such a small part of my body, I wonder what else the smoke did to me both externally and internally.

Smoker's Cough

Inside our wonderful lungs are small hair-like villi that normally clean foreign matter from the lungs by "waving" the contaminant out of the lungs, where it is swallowed and then disposed of by the body. These villi are stunted when you smoke and so you no longer have this normal, natural cleaning system working in your favor. The only way that your lungs can dispose of any contaminant or mucous is by incorporating the "coughing mechanism." By the way, the number of contaminants in smoke is too great to discuss here. Years ago, nicotine was used to poison coyotes out in the western part of the U.S.

Coughing is not easy on the body as demonstrated by older, frail people sometimes fracturing a rib by the extreme motion of coughing. You *have* to cough to get rid of this junk that you have been putting into your lungs for years. It is so unpleasant to hear a constant smoker's cough because you know that this is a self-inflicted situation, and almost the entire world knows the damage of smoking to anyone's body. I have had patients who have lost both parents and other relatives to lung cancer and know very well that their long-term smoking was the major cause of their painful death, but the patient is still smoking! After talking to this patient one day about her continued smoking, I reexamined her chart and was amazed that she looked 20 years older than her chronological age! I thought it might just be my inability to judge age appropriately, so I waited until she had left and then asked the employees up front how old they thought she was. They also guessed 20 years older than her real age. As a provider you put into this patient's chart "appears older than stated age." This is not a good thing to have said about you, but in this case the patient had such a severe "smoker's mask," it aged her two decades.

I have had smokers on constant oxygen due to smoking who still smoke! One younger man forgot to remove his oxygen nasal cannula before lighting up and wound up in the ER due to the explosion that burned him badly enough to leave scars and caused immediate loss of facial hair and the front part of the hair on his scalp. He still smokes!

The good news is that when you totally stop smoking, these cleansing villi in the lungs regenerate in about three to four months. So even after you are successful in stopping totally, you will still need to use the coughing mechanism to clear the lungs for several months.

I want to leave this section on nicotine with the original question: "Why do you need this terribly addictive drug in this wonderful body you have?" Forgive me for being so very basic, but this is such an important part of your life to overcome. You *know* you should not smoke or use any tobacco products. When it is so obvious to you that you need to stop smoking but you have not, the excuses sound so empty that you may be ashamed to even admit to yourself or others that you still are addicted to nicotine.

Caffeine

Now I am really stepping into territory that makes others uncomfortable! We should start with "Why do I need caffeine?" Well, why **do** you need caffeine? Are you aware you can really live without it? Some of my seminar participants reply, "Why should we want to live without caffeine?" I realize that many will stop reading or attempting to understand now that I am talking about something as universally consumed as caffeine. We need to continue to ask ourselves what is going on in our lives that we need caffeine to get started.

Please bear with me as I attempt to describe this situation. You have been asleep for hours. Your body has lost a great deal of water by the normal loss of water during breathing and evaporation. Your stomach acid is higher than at just about any other time during the day without having food in it to digest. You awaken without being refreshed, and the absolute first thing to hit this wonderful body you have been given is a super jolt of acidic coffee or an acidic, carbonated, caffeine-laced drink! The only worse thing you can do to your body is to start smoking a cigarette and hit your brain with a nicotine jolt. Ask yourself, is that really *good* for your body? Would you allow your children to do that when they were young? Do you advise your children to do that as they mature? Now it is time to reevaluate why you do this to your body.

I implore you to start protecting this wonderful body you not only live in now but will for the rest of your life! The body is AMAZING! But we often mistreat it for years and then wonder why it begins to fail us later in life. It is extremely sad to talk to patients who are remorseful that they treated their bodies so badly earlier in their lives. The body has a wonderful capacity to compensate for such inappropriate treatment and can do so for years, but then several systems begin to "fatigue" at approximately the same time and then you begin to plan your life around visits to healthcare providers of all specialties rather than enjoying your later years. Most of us are blessed with good health when younger (with some exceptions, of course) but way too many with good health "self-inflict" damage on our bodies to cause misery later in life that cannot be undone even if the unhealthy habits are broken.

Caffeine is a stimulant...why do you need a stimulant? Why every day? Why many times a day or even all day long? When your body is in its natural state, you don't need caffeine. We need to change our lifestyle so this is not a "need" of our bodies to function.

We will be discussing adequate sleep soon, but for now, reexamine your life to consider why you need a stimulant at any time and also why the greatest need may be in the morning. I remember when I drank coffee nearly all day long (I still miss drinking coffee after thirty-five years of not drinking any). I would have a caffeine "high" and then I would experience a "down" feeling as the caffeine concentration diminished, and I would then drink more caffeine to reverse this trend. So all day long I was up and down. When I finally stopped drinking caffeine totally (not even decaffeinated drinks), my mood (which significantly affects your life) was level all day, every day. This was a tremendous benefit to me and probably also my family. I drank that much coffee because I had read that caffeine could help with migraines, but when I stopped, they did not get any worse or improve either.

Caffeine is in so many products now that it is almost impossible to avoid. Some pain medicines have a great deal of caffeine even if over the counter. One of the most popular soft drinks is Mountain

Dew®, which has been a wonderful financial success. When I was working in the ER in a nearby hospital, there was an article in the local newspaper about how Mountain Dew had been developed in this small town as a cocktail mix. It was discovered and aggressively marketed by a major beverage company; it is for sale everywhere it seems. It was always the drink of choice of my patients because they would drag their large bottles of warm Mountain Dew into my office, knowing that I was going to scold them about not drinking water. If you ever want to see the impact of this drink on teeth, just search YouTube for experiments about it. The dentists now have a diagnosis called "Dew mouth" because of the damage it does to teeth. Other drinks do also, but since Mountain Dew is so prevalent, it gets most of the blame. Dental caries (cavities) is one of the most prevalent problems of the Native Americans in remote villages in Alaska; they fly the powered drinks in because it is too expensive to fly the full drink in.

The new trend of "energy" drinks is troubling! They are so full of caffeine and sugar that they will give you energy, but it is false energy and not from a natural process that works with your body to also give you a natural "high." One of my dearest friends, who is very stressed due to his successful healthcare business, opened one of the small bottles of very concentrated sugar and caffeine and drank it as we talked. I hated that for him because he has so very much to offer the healthcare world, and I don't want him to do anything to lessen his very considerable ability.

Caffeine is most often in chocolate, so that may be why people like chocolate so much. Another thing to consider when you are eating chocolate is that most of what you are eating are paraffin-type products with the chocolate mixed in, so now your body has to process a foreign substance that has no value to the body. I enjoy chocolate for the taste, but even the small amount that I eat (most of the time) has enough caffeine to "wire" me for several hours since

I am not accustomed to caffeine anymore.

When you stop caffeine consumption, you will feel very bad for a few days as I did when I stopped on Thanksgiving morning about thirty-five years ago. I chose a long weekend just to deal with the withdrawal, and it was a good thing that I did. I have never regretted that decision and am pleased every day that I was able to do so. I am still in excellent health for an older person and take no prescription or OTC meds with the exception of some antihistamines (Claritin®) during my worst allergy season in the spring. I know I have been blessed with good health, but I have also kept most harmful substances out of my body. That is such a benefit to me, and I want you to have the opportunity to experience the same good feeling even if you have to endure some withdrawal symptoms. When you know you are doing right by your body, there is a peace because you know that you are not doing harm to it. Caffeine is harmful to the body!

Sugar

If caffeine is everywhere, sugar (processed sugar) is even worse! It is even in the toothpaste you are using to prevent cavities! That was a revelation to me. For years I lectured on nutrition as a part of my work with DuPont, so I was able to study this subject while I was getting paid, plus I had access to any literature reference I wanted because they had a service to provide that for me. I started focusing on the sugar content listed on the label that is required on all food. You will find (most often) sugars listed under different names, because if they were all lumped together, sugar would often be the first ingredient on the list. The government requires that the larger volumes of ingredients be listed first, down to the least volume. Different names for sugar include brown sugar, fructose, sucrose, molasses, corn syrup, honey, and chocolate sugar. This is very concerning! Why do they break the sugars up? Mostly so you will not be able to determine how much the sugar content actually is.

One of the presentations I did while in my medical training was to research how much sugar really is in certain foods. Tomato catsup is over 20% sugar, dark chocolate brownies are over 50%, and even Weight Watcher's energy bars have sugar in them at varying amounts. I was so disappointed to find that one of my favorite treats of a large Frosty® (chocolate, of course) has over 900 calories! The larger milkshakes are nearly 1,000 calories, and some are even more if you add whipped cream or other toppings.

These high levels of sugar in our drinks and foods have been implicated in our increasing obesity and diabetes problems. So, if you eat a normal amount of food to satisfy your feeling of hunger, the foods you eat may be so full of sugar that it puts you well over the number of calories to maintain your weight. Now, if you eat more food than you really need, you are just compounding the problems. Our children's food is often heavily sugar concentrated to get them to eat it, just as the sugar in toothpaste will give them a better feeling about brushing their teeth.

Even the sugar substitutes are being implicated in diabetes because they make your body <u>think</u> it has the full sugar load. I had a family practice clinic in one of the lower economic areas of town (I purposely had a clinic there), and right across the street were two very busy convenience stores. As you have experienced, most of the walls of these stores are lined with refrigerated display cases. In the busiest store there was not even one diet beverage available, and the other store had only one small line of diet beverages and almost no water.

We are now back to the same question of why do we need that sugar? Sugar will give you an upswing in energy, but it will also cause a downswing later—so the net gain is nothing, but the damage to your body is something to consider once again. YOU can live without processed sugars. If you like a sweet dessert after a meal, the very best thing to eat is a sweet fruit, and there are many that will give you the same taste but without the processed sugar content.

Additives/Preservatives

There are certain foods that have more additives and preservatives than others, so as we attempt to keep our bodies from having to deal with too much and too many other substances, we might consider some of these foods. The one that first comes to mind for me is pepperoni. Unfortunately, I really like pepperoni on pizza, but every time I eat one of those wonderful-tasting circles, I wonder what all the additives in this food are that preserve it for so long and what is it doing to me. So, just look at what you are eating to minimize the level of additives and preservatives you eat.

Fruit for Breakfast

There is a surefire way you can get natural energy that is totally good for your body when you awaken in the mornings! When you eat fruit and your stomach is empty (as it should be after a night's sleep) the fruit is processed very quickly if you *only* eat fruit. The fruit leaves the stomach and goes into the small intestine quickly. Any food only gives the body energy when it is processed in the small intestine. If your stomach is empty and you eat only natural fruit, it moves into the small intestine in approximately thirty minutes. Bananas, America's favorite fruit, take closer to forty-five minutes.

If you eat the fruit with other types of foods, then the fruit is digested at the same time the other foods are processed and does not progress into the small intestine until it all begins to move there. If you want to be good to your wonderful body, then feed it natural fruit the very first thing rather than jolting it awake with acidic drinks that contain caffeine. This may delay your quick energy for about thirty minutes, but it is so much better for your body, and it will start your day in a natural way, especially if you have already drank enough water to experience the cascade of coolness.

There is another benefit that may be important to you. Fruit seems to be a natural stimulant for the innermost sphincter in the rectum, which allows the fecal material to move from the large intestine into position behind the outermost sphincter that you control for defecation. The body controls the innermost sphincter to give you the urge to defecate, but thankfully, we are in control of the outermost one.

Picture your stomach when you put natural fruit into it—it now has only one type of food to process, and it is food that is excellent for the body in addition to providing you with relatively quick, natural energy! When we eat other types of foods first, it takes several hours before we get any energy production, plus the digestion of the food requires energy from what you ate the night before. You can eat other breakfast food later, before you leave home, as long as you allow the body to process the natural fruit first.

Fruit is reasonably inexpensive, easy to keep, and requires no cooking; it can be eaten while driving (if necessary), and the cleanup is very easy. You may need to do this for a few days before your body adjusts, but the reward is well worth the effort. If you only eat fruit for breakfast, then your snack at mid-morning could also be fruit. Once you start this simple, natural program, you may want to have some days where you eat more fruit (by itself) for lunch. This is a simple request where you use natural foods to put into your natural body based on the knowledge of how fruit moves quickly into the "energy room" (small intestine)—so what could be wrong about this suggestion?

Do You Need to Lose Weight?

I ask this question because it is one that I have to deal with, along with most people today. Drinking water, reducing or eliminating sugared drinks, eating natural foods as often as possible—this is a wonderful start. If you add a routine exercise program, you should have a better chance of maintaining your desired weight. I have never had a real problem with weight, but I don't like myself very well when my clothing becomes tighter than before.

If you do need to lose weight, then in my opinion there is one word for it—Atkins, or any high-protein, low-carbohydrate diet. I used to attend national conventions of the American Dieticians Society groups on how to recognize malnutrition in hospitalized patients. These folks are serious about their diet! It was so good to be a part of some of their programs. There were very few obese attendees at these conventions! Normally, when I would go to a convention I did not have much problem using whatever exercise equipment the hotel provided...except if it was a convention of dietitians. They were all over that equipment, so I would often just have to run outside. One time I had forgotten to pack my running shoes, so I just ran on the treadmill in my socks. Several people saw me later in the day to ask me if that was a new trend in exercising, so they even paid attention to anything that could be a new happening in exercise.

They nearly always allowed discussion in the sessions about different dietetic topics. It was amazing what a fire storm I would cause when I would mention the Atkins diet! At times I felt in danger for my life! After everyone had told me why it would not work and was very damaging to the body, I would ask how many of them had even read the book. Nearly always the answer was that they had not read it because they just knew it would not work and would raise your cholesterol from the protein. Then my next question would be if they knew of any research why it would <u>not</u> work. Silence. Now, there has been research that the high-protein, low-carb diet does not damage the body nor raise cholesterol. When I need to lose a few pounds, I switch into this mode, and I do that because it works! One of the biggest benefits of this diet is that it takes away my craving for sweets. That is a wonderful benefit that is supposed to be due to the low carbs, because eating carbs causes the body to desire more carbs.

You only eat nearly all protein for about two weeks, and then you start adding in other foods that have natural carbs. You will not die during the first two weeks! Often it is reported that people's energy level increases because of not dealing with carbs. I sometimes attended a morning breakfast meeting at a pancake restaurant. I would eat protein but also have a couple of pancakes with no-sugar-added syrup. I began to notice that on those days when I ate there at about 8 AM, by 4 PM I felt like I had completely run out of gas and had a difficult time focusing on my work for the next few hours due to the lack of energy. I still go to the breakfast meeting, but I don't eat the pancakes anymore and I no longer have the afternoon drop of energy.

Protein-rich foods are a little more expensive, but you can save money by not feeling the hunger for the snacks that are usually sugar- and carb-heavy. If I eat a hearty protein breakfast, I most often don't even feel any hunger at lunch and just keep working or rest. If you have never tried this type of diet, I suggest you do so. You will know within two weeks if it will benefit you. As always, keep drinking a great deal of water. You will notice some small changes within a few weeks, sometimes even within the two-week period. If you exercise, you will notice more changes. Your clothing may not be quite as tight, or you may notice some loss of weight in your fingers and hands. That is where I notice it first, even without having fat fingers normally. When I have the chance to suture lacerations (cuts) on patients' fingers, I am always surprised how much adipose (fat) tissue there is, even in slender fingers. Sometimes you can't get all of it back under the skin, so you just remove it without any damage to the finger. It is good to notice changes quickly because you will know that the plan is working! You will feel better about yourself very quickly, and you will know that you are on a good path toward achieving your goal. I am certain that there are other diet plans that work, but this one works best for me.

If you stay on a reasonably high-protein diet, you will find that the weight is more apt to say off, and you will not "yo-yo." Adipose cells are uniquely shaped in that they appear to be a slightly yellow "baggie" with the nucleus over to the side, whereas most other body cells' nuclei are somewhat centered in the cell tissue. The fat cells can grow much bigger than their nucleus appears to be able to support. Unfortunately, when you lose weight the baggie remains, so it is easier for the body to fill it up again than to make a new one.

I use visual imaging to help me with this weight loss process. I picture several little men in tall rubber boots who go around to the fat cells and pierce them with long spears to allow the fat to escape, which is why they wear the tall rubber boots... This imagery does amuse me, so I think of it often and sometimes even give the fat-piercing workers suggestions of where to work today. It seems that I most often tell them to focus on my waist area, but I am not convinced that my communication is successful. When you notice other places than your hands, it will be interesting to see where you can notice the fat reduction next. One place for me is the outside muscle on my upper arm. It now is more visible, so that tells me that

I am being somewhat successful. I do envy those with a six-pack, but I am not willing to work that hard.

If you want to appear less overweight, just purchase clothing that fits. For instance, in men, for approximately every eight to ten pounds you gain, your shirt neck size increases a half size. So if it is difficult to button your shirt at the neck and you have gained ten to twenty pounds, then it is time to change shirt sizes. Even the sleeve length is affected as you gain weight because the measurement for a man's sleeve length is from the center of the neck to the wrist, and if you have gained weight, some of it will be on your back, thereby increasing the shirt sleeve length.

Clothing that fits appropriately helps reduce your stress greatly! If something is too small, it reveals some of the bulges that you may not find attractive. For men, wearing clothes that are too tight at the waist could impact the digestive system somewhat by restricting the normal amount of room. If when you take your shoes off it seems that your feet have been holding their breath all day, then it is time to move to a larger size. My heart goes out to women because it seems that they have such a problem finding shoes that both look good and feel good. I have heard that women usually gain a shoe size with each of their first few pregnancies.

Fat

We have become overly obsessed with the amount of fat in our diets due to the concerns of high cholesterol levels that can cause a heart attack or stroke. It is often amazing to see a young athletic man or woman with high cholesterol, and it is very surprising to them. Your body makes about half the cholesterol it has, so attempting to lower high cholesterol with diet is seldom successful enough unless the person maintains an aggressive exercise program. The professors told us in our medical training that diet only lowers the cholesterol level about 15-20%, and often that is not enough. Again, the very best way to handle this is to diet, even if it only contributes 15%, and to implement a good exercise routine, which is best for us anyway. I found that few patients were willing to exercise and/or diet sufficiently, so I would start them on a cholesterol-lowering drug with the hope of reducing or eliminating the medicines as soon as possible. The danger of not controlling the high cholesterol is greater than the side effects of the medicines in most cases.

With the high-protein diet, your cholesterol levels will actually decrease, which is contrary to what you would think since you are adding more fat to the diet. I have had this proven on my own patients when they switch to the Atkins-type diet. I understand that the popular Dr. Oz calls this the caveman diet. Try it for yourself before you discount it.

Adequate Sleep

I think sleep is such a fascinating subject. One minute you are awake and the next microsecond you are in la la land! This is truly a major transition in your body. Have you ever observed a child who has gone to sleep while eating a cookie? Do you remember the last time you drove an automobile and had some "micro-sleep" seconds when everything became really quiet even if the radio was blaring in your attempt to stay awake? That is such a frightening moment that just the adrenaline of the incident will keep you awake, but only for a short time.

If you want to <u>put</u> someone to sleep, it requires either some rather serious trauma to their head or very strong chemicals that cause the body to go into a sleep state. I have studied sleep for years because of my fascination with it. Fortunately, now there is a great deal of research due to so many sleep studies being performed routinely.

There is one fundamental fact about sleep that can help you understand this process better. You cannot sleep more than your body needs, nor can you "store up" sleep time to use later. If you are sleeping more now, it may very well be due to the fact that you need more sleep and/or you may have another medical problem like depression, low hormone levels, or even stress that is not controlled adequately. So a good physical exam with laboratory testing may be in order—ask for it before someone starts giving you sleep medicines. There are medicines that can help you sleep, but most are for only short-term use, and if they keep working for you for many months or years, then you may be only getting the placebo effect, where your body just thinks it is getting benefit from the medicine.

Sleep deprivation is very hard on our bodies and is used sometimes to make prisoners of war talk by not allowing them to go to sleep for days. Of course, the statements they make in sleep deprivation may be nonsensical. Much of our society is sleep-deprived! Fortunately, again, there is a natural way for you to determine if you are getting adequate sleep unless there are some medical problems in addition to deal with. Our brain has an internal clock that works wonderfully and so well that some people do not find it necessary to even set an alarm. ("Alarm" is certainly a negative term to have to consider when you are attempting to awaken!) Your wonderful brain will awaken you ten to fifteen minutes prior to just about any alarm *if* you have adequate rest. I often set an alarm in case I am more tired than I thought, but nearly always I awaken prior to the alarm clock shocking me from sleep, as many use the alarm to do. In a more inventive time of my life, I attempted to design an alarm clock that you could throw and smash into pieces so you could 1. Silence the ALARM and 2. Get any pent-up aggression out of the way before the day even started! I thought it might be a big seller, but I kept having a problem putting it back together so it would function properly the next day.

Those who study brain wave functions relate that when you awaken before the alarm and before you actually start moving your body is the time when the communication between the two halves (hemispheres) of the brain is the greatest and the creative part of the brain and the physical part are their most productive and interactive. I have found that this appears to be true in my life. It is so pleasant to awaken normally, somewhat refreshed, and lie there to contemplate the day or even better to meditate. If your meditation puts you back to sleep, then the alarm will awaken you.

Bottom line of sleep adequacy—if you have to awaken nearly every day to the alarm, then you are not getting enough sleep. What is the process of correcting this problem? Get more sleep! When you are driving a one- to two-ton vehicle and you are sleepy, then there is really only one solution...stop and get some sleep. Caffeine, loud music, cold air blowing on your face will not be sufficient unless you are very, very close to your destination. Certainly, when you are sleepy, it is no time to use cruise control on your car.

I remember meeting a couple whose young son was totally paralyzed due to a tragic automobile accident. The father was driving and told the mother that he was going to stop at the next exit to rest because he was getting too sleepy to drive. She was preparing their son for the stop and took the restraints off their child, and the father went to sleep as he was driving down the exit ramp. The ensuing accident meant that now, every day, they have to take care of their son's most basic needs due to their mutual mistakes.

There are so many things that attempt (or tempt us) to keep us awake. Our instant communication abilities work against our getting adequate sleep. How many times have you been surprised when you have checked some news program (all bad news), your email, Facebook, YouTube, or whatever grabs your attention and then you realize that you have spent a great deal more time there than you planned? I have certainly done that. In just the last day or so I went to bed early but awakened at about three AM. I thought I would respond to a "friend request" and received a response back in about ten minutes. She was a new mother and was awake for the early morning feeding, so that amused me greatly because they love having this newborn in their home.

I have had so many patients request sleep medications because they can't go to sleep. Certainly before you give someone a medicine that only works for a short time, you need to ask some basic questions. The first is "Do you smoke?" Remember, over 80% of my patients smoke, so the answer is almost always yes. Then I ask if they smoke just prior to going to bed and/or do they smoke when they awaken during the night. Most of the time the answer is yes to both! So many have expressed surprise that appears to be genuine when I tell them that nicotine is a very powerful stimulant that I begin to wonder if they really don't know that nicotine can keep them awake. Keep in mind that most of my patients don't read. Most can read but they just don't read, and nearly all the information they get is from verbal conversations and/or TV type of media.

Then I ask them if they take any caffeine prior to going to sleep, and again the most common answer is yes. I tell them that caffeine has a six-hour half-life (which means six hours later, half of the stimulant power is gone but the other half is still there!), so taking in any caffeine can keep them awake. I tell them to use Benadryl or some OTC drug because I will not prescribe sleep meds if they are using strong stimulants prior to going to sleep.

If you can smoke and/or take caffeine and still go to sleep, then take that as a serious warning sign that you are certainly sleep-deprived! If your body is fatigued enough that you can go to sleep after strong stimulants, then you will not sleep long or deep enough to get restorative sleep. Your body may go to sleep temporarily, but the stimulants will awaken you before you get what sleep you need even if you have been practicing this habit for years.

It appears that if you have to use the alarm to awaken most of the time, initially you need to go to sleep ninety minutes or an hour and a half earlier than your usual routine until your body gets the proper amount of rest it needs. After you are no longer in sleep deprivation, you may find that you can shorten this time of early retirement. Your signal that you are getting out of your sleep-deprived state will be when you begin to awaken several minutes prior to the alarm because, remember, you can't sleep longer than your body needs in most cases. If you can get adequate sleep, your mornings will be much more pleasant for you and others around you. You will awaken prior to an "ugly" alarm, have a few minutes of quiet time to meditate or plan your day, drink water until you feel the cascade of coolness, and eat some fresh fruit for natural, healthy energy to start your day off positively. Now that you are getting adequate sleep, you feel better in the morning, and you can tolerate the thirty minutes or so before the fruit begins to "kick in," so your day can be more natural without stimulants.

Sleep Hygiene

Again, this new emphasis on sleep research has allowed healthcare providers to establish a routine for going to sleep that has been validated many times. It is called "sleep hygiene" and has simple, basic suggestions to help your body transition into the sleep state when you want it to. It starts with a set time to go to sleep if you can arrange your life to allow for that most of the time. Then you have a routine of your body's actions telling your brain that you are preparing for "sleepy time" now. That routine may be to brush your teeth, put on (or take off) whatever clothing you normally sleep in, and then get into bed. Another "mind management" process that seems to help most people is to begin listing all the positive things in their life for that day and not allowing their thoughts to go negative.

One requirement is no TV or media devices in the bedroom, period! The bedroom is to be limited to two activities, and both of them start with the letter "s." Sleep is the first one, and sex is the other one. Sex, while stimulating, if satisfying, can lead to better sleep.

TV is not designed to help you sleep, ever! It is designed to keep you awake so you can buy more stuff! It has flashing lights and exciting commercials to keep you awake so you can be exposed to more commercials. Even the previews to the next show are often the best part of the entire show, so you have just wasted another hour of sleep or real rest time thinking this was going to be a good use of your time. But after it is over, you may think that preview was the only part of the show worth watching. You may think you can go

SLEEP HYGIENE

to sleep better with the TV on, and hopefully that is not true, which means you have been doing that for years, and also for years your wonderful brain has listened to millions of commercials and heard bad news for hours while you were attempting to get restorative sleep! That is horrible! Your brain hears all of that, and even your eyes can see the changes in the light intensity through the eyelids even if you turn your head away from the screen. Do yourself a huge favor and get the TV completely out of the bedroom, immediately, or it will not happen.

What happens if you go to bed and can't go to sleep? First examine what you have consumed the last several hours to see if any stimulants have impacted your ability to go to sleep. Eliminate them as soon as possible. Sleep research has demonstrated that if you don't go to sleep in the first twenty minutes of going to bed, you become frustrated and can even become angry at your body because it will NOT go to sleep! After twenty minutes with no sleep, get out of bed and go to a quiet place and read nonstimulating reading material like this book or magazines or self-help or spiritual material until you become sleepy. I don't need to mention here that you are not to watch TV or exciting movies. Now that you feel sleepy, go back to bed. If you have another twenty minutes with no success in bed, then go back to the quiet place and continue repeating this process until you do get sleepy enough to sleep in your bed. Sleep research has also demonstrated that men and women have different sleep patterns. Generally men go into their deeper and restorative sleep early in the sleep time, and women get their restorative sleep more toward the end of the sleep time. We all have different needs for sleep. Let's assume that both men and women need eight hours of sleep. If they both only get six hours, it will be more damaging to the woman because her more restorative sleep time will be shortened or eliminated, whereas the man has already received most of their restorative sleep. In many homes the woman gets less sleep than the man, so she has less good sleep time and that can begin to affect her health. So if you are female, please be aware of these sleep pattern differences, explain them to any men who might need to be enlightened, and go to sleep!

This difference in sleep patterns is why some question if women will be as successful as men in combat situations. It does not speak to any difference in bravery or intelligence but only the fundamental needs of the body. The hard-core rules of combat are when combat is over you do three things as soon as possible. Clean your weapon and make sure you have adequate ammunition. Then you eat so you will have energy. Then you go to sleep even if it is the middle of the day because you don't know when you will have another chance to sleep if you need to go back into combat. If there is a prolonged time of short sleep sessions due to the ongoing combat situation, then it will negatively impact the woman more than the man due to the fundamental sleep patterns of gaining restorative sleep.

If you have children, it is very important that they get adequate sleep. Teenagers and preteens need the same amount of sleep that toddlers do to feel refreshed. Their bodies are using a great deal of energy in the changing and growing process, so they need a good deal of sleep as well as extra calories. It is not good to allow them to get into adult habits of inadequate sleep and then stimulating the body to attempt to function properly.

This is such a simple problem that we all face at times, but it is critical that we get adequate sleep! If this is a problem for you, please attempt the natural suggestions mentioned here before resorting to any artificial substances to achieve a restive sleep state. Regular exercise will also help you sleep even if it is close to your bedtime.

Reduce TV

If you want to reduce your stress level, reduce your exposure to TV. It is that simple, but few are willing to do this. Keep in mind that I am so convinced that the suggestions here will help you that I will give you your money back if you practice them for thirty days and your stress level does not go down. This one suggestion just by itself is almost enough to justify a money-back guarantee!

Why do we allow this method of communicating to invade our personal space for so many hours each and every day? <u>Really</u>, why do we do that? Do we need all that negative information over and over for hours every day for most of our lives? I know this is a serious challenge, but it is a fundamental question of how to help you do better with stress, avoid stress-related problems, and live a happier life. That is quite a package of positive benefits for just one simple task of reducing the media access to your life.

If you do this for thirty days, you will realize what an unhealthy practice we have been fooled into thinking that TV has a right to invade our privacy. If you do want to watch one of the programs, and there are many good ones, then watch it, but don't be lured into "staying tuned" for what is next. Please control the TV rather than letting it control you. You will be amazed by the peace and calmness in your personal space when you isolate yourself from this bombardment of mostly useless, negative information. Also, don't get caught up into the habit of hearing all the "bad news" before going to bed or before starting your day. It is amazing how many hours we are exposed to sensational cases that have happened in far parts of the U.S. or even other parts of the world.

Time Management to Reduce Stress—Leave Early

I used to have the habit of working or doing something until the very last minute before leaving for a meeting or anything that required being on time, like work. Then I had to hit every traffic signal just perfectly, I had no time to allow for traffic problems, and I arrived wherever I was going stressed—when all I had to do to minimize this problem was to leave just a few minutes earlier. I am ashamed to say it was that simple. Now, if you are early, you can at least text someone or check your email even if you are where you cannot carry on a verbal conversation.

Do this for thirty days and soon into your change you will see that this is a serious stress reducer. I even recommend that you put your seat belt on before your automobile beeps at you because to me it is not pleasant to have someone (or even worse *something*) telling me that I need to do something. I also used to drive as fast as I could without getting a traffic ticket. I have dropped that habit because now I am much less stressed by being concerned about another ticket.

Use your new electronic toys to plan your work and life because if you have your tasks in your planner, then you don't have to retain them in your mind and keep wondering if you are "on track." Our new technology is wonderful if used correctly and can actually assist in reducing stress, so look for that part of any device you have access to.

Dictation Technology

One of the better uses of technology to reduce stress is to use some manner of dictating. It is amazing how this can reduce your stress because it takes away the concern of what you need to do. All it takes is a quick verbal note to yourself like "Don't forget to have Mr. X call Ms. Y about budget." Of course you must retrieve the messages on a regular basis or the benefit is too late. If you can get someone else to take off the notes for you at work, that is an even better use of your time. You can even speed it up if you have a specific message for someone by using their name at the beginning of your recording so you will know to put that chore on the other person's list rather than yours.

You may have a wonderful idea or remember something important enough to write down, but you are driving and, if you are like me, by the time you exit and park safely enough to write something down, you will have forgotten what it was. Now you are even more frustrated. I even keep my recorder by my bed at night in case of a good thought coming along as I awaken during the night or even the next morning when I am in that creative time of the day. You can do that without having to turn the light on or get into a position that would allow you to write your thought down. I keep the device on my desk in case I am in the middle of some project that I might have to close or save to get to my computer calendar or list of projects.

Speaking of lists, if you want to really become productive, use a daily list of projects to accomplish. It feels so good to be able to draw a line through a project that sometimes if I have accomplished something that was not on my list, I write it on the list so I can draw a line through it! This gives me some sense of accomplishment for that day to offset the ones that I have to keep on my to-do list. Managing this list is very important, and using a recording device can make the entire process much easier and thereby reduce your stress.

One other management benefit, if you are managing any other employees, is to put the responsibility on them to follow up with you and keep you informed about their progress rather than you having to go to them to check on their progress. This will take some doing, but it will reduce your mental effort of tracking projects you have assigned to your employees. If they encounter a problem, they should inform you of the problem and have suggested solutions already for your review. This frees you up to do other important projects because you have achieved some level of success or you would not have others reporting to you.

Cell Phone

What a wonderful invention! This can both reduce your stress and also increase your stress if you allow others to abuse your time because they know you have a cell phone. I continue to be amazed by how we as a society have allowed the cell phone to change our lives even for the negative. Some people are very stressed because they feel it is their responsibility to be available at any time and every call is important. The call may be important to the person making it, but it does not mean that it is important to you. We have allowed others to invade our privacy and "peace time" by responding or at least looking to see who is calling even if we do not answer the call.

I have found that my life goes along very well if I reduce the invasion of my life. When I am at home resting, either by going to sleep or just attempting to be at peace, I just turn off both the house and cell phones. This does not create a problem because both have answering capabilities and I can return calls later. I love that anonymous quote, "Poor planning on your part does not constitute an emergency on my part!" I have a very elderly father, but I know that if he passes away, there is someone or some agency to help, so it is okay for me to miss a few hours of being connected. All my family members have the phone numbers of my immediate neighbors to use in an extreme emergency, or if it is an even greater emergency the local law enforcement agencies will respond. I have done this for years and have yet to miss anything that had to be seen about (by me) immediately.

I always wondered what would happen if someone in my family had an accident and needed me. They have had several accidents over the years, and there has always been someone to take care of their immediate need. One morning my granddaughter had an accident while with her father. Fortunately neither of them was hurt, but he had some legal issues that were brought to light by the responding officers and was escorted away to attend to those issues. A mother stopped and saw what was happening, and she went into that wonderful "I will take care of this" mode. She called my daughter to tell her of the situation, and then let my granddaughter talk to her mother. Then she took my granddaughter to her school and allowed her to talk to her mother the entire way. This mother took care of my granddaughter and went out of her way to take her to another school, even while making her children late to their own school.

We need to gain all the benefit from our emerging technology while realizing that there is a downside, and it must be controlled if it is increasing our stress level. Our health is more important than most, if not all, the messages we receive. We delete most emails anyway, so why should we feel that we need to check them so continuously?

Music—Classical Reduces Beta-Endorphins

Music can be very relaxing, and commercials can be very stressful, as can the news. There are times when we need no outside stimulation, and we need to relish those moments and use them to de-stress. We discussed earlier the benefit of classical music reducing the level of stress substances (beta-endorphins). This research was reported in the article "The effect of selected classical music and spontaneous imagery on plasma beta-endorphin" in the Journal of Behavioral Medicine. 1977 Feb:20(1). 85-99. by McKinney, Tims, Kumar and Kumar. My dentist spends a great deal of time and money selecting this type of music to assist his patients and staff in being relaxed. He is an excellent dentist and friend and totally minimizes the stress of going to a dentist, which is always high on the list of unpleasant activities for most people.

There are times when upbeat music can be therapeutic in elevating your mood and thereby lowering your stress level, but continued listening to more and more exciting music can cause even more stress because you are continuing to look for music that will do an even better job of elevating your mood.

Audio Books

This is a great way to reduce stress because it allows you to "read" something that you might never have time to otherwise. You feel like you are still learning while driving rather than only driving. I have listened to books that I might not ever taken the time to read. You will be amazed how much "reading" you can do while you are driving. It can even take some of the stress off of your driving if it is a good book, as long as it does not distract you.

Safety

You may be wondering what "safety" is doing in a stress reduction book! Safety consciousness has a tremendous impact on your stress level. If you think you are stressed right now, what would it do to your stress level if you were now on crutches on in a cast or anything that needed enough immediate attention to cause your stress level to increase? Also being very stressed can lead to accidents that cause even more stress.

I was so very fortunate to work for a company that taught safety strategies to all employees to use at work and at home. They were self-insured the twenty-plus years I worked for them, so every accident cost them money for medical care as well as lost productivity. DuPont has an excellent safety record, one of the best in the world, and they even have a part of their business to teach other companies to be safer. The money to purchase these courses is offset by the buyer because of the overall cost savings of focusing on safety, so I am back to this: If business thinks something is good for business, then it may very well be good for us also.

We are often cautious about our family members' safety but fail to protect ourselves; if we are injured, then those around us suffer from the consequences if not from the actual pain. DuPont paid for safety glasses to use at home and even steel-toed shoes to use if you were mowing your lawn. It was required that you hold onto a handrail anytime you went up or down stairs. All hot beverage containers had to have a lid if you were walking with them. Seat belts must be worn at all times in an automobile, and you could (and would) be fired if you were driving a company vehicle without a seat belt on and you had an accident. They also rewarded you if you and your office or factory were safe for a certain time. These awards were useful and it was almost like Christmas when the safety prize catalog came in the mail.

Safety was so prevalent that if I were taking someone somewhere and I was using my company car and they refused to wear a seat belt, then I would park my car and take another means of transportation. The one "not my fault" accident I had was one that could have been a big problem for my passenger. We had been to see some equipment that she was considering purchasing and were returning to her hospital. I had made her wear her seat belt all day because she was not accustomed to doing so. As we were stopped at a traffic light, she was leaning over to pick up some literature that I had given her, and she started to unfasten her seat belt. Then she looked at me and laughed and said, "I almost took this off." Just then I noticed a car approaching at a high rate of speed in the rearview mirror, and I began to accelerate to avoid the impact even with the traffic light was still red because I had checked to see that nothing was coming from the left or right. The elderly lady who hit us in the rear never even touched her brakes, and the impact totaled my company car. My passenger and I were only shaken up, but she would have been injured very badly if she had not left her seat belt on. I ask you to please put your seat belt on even before you begin driving rather than put it on later as you begin your drive.

If you are involved in sports, please attempt to reduce your chances of an accident, and protect yourself as best as you can if you do have one. Always wear eye protection when painting the ceiling or even the wall or when using a power tool either inside the house or outside in the yard. You will never regret holding onto the rail on stairs, but you will certainly regret when you fall either going up or down and you did not do something as simple as keeping your hand on the rail. Do this for yourself as well as for others. It is a wonderful, lifetime attitude to be aware of safety and can significantly reduce your stress.

Driving an automobile right now is more dangerous than it has ever been! We forget how dangerous an automobile accident can be until someone we know has a serious accident. I have seen so many young people who have life-damaging scars and changes to their body due to an accident, and most often they were not wearing a seat belt.

Drivers are distracted now, cars are quieter so you do not realize how fast you are going, and many put too much reliance on anti-locking brakes and airbags to protect them. In addition, so many drivers are sleep-deprived that the "micro-sleep" state can be deadly.

I have had twelve full days of nothing but driving safety during my career. These are eight to five, all day behind the wheel or observing someone else drive. Often these courses are expensive to attend and even require travel expense. I thought I knew how to drive because I had my own car at age fifteen and had been driving for a year before that on my own. I was so wrong! There is so much to learn about safe driving, and I always learned something useful even on the last days of these courses where you would have thought you had time to learn everything.

The main thing is to keep a big "bubble" around you to allow for your mistakes as well as the other driver so you can avoid an accident. I can't tell you how many times this bubble has saved me from an accident. Also be aware of all cars around you at all times so you can make a quick change to a safety zone rather than having to look to make the change when danger is imminent. If you start looking into your mirror more when driving on the interstate, you will notice that often you are all alone! There will be a pack of cars ahead and behind, but you will be totally alone or almost so. This is something that amazed me—how often it happens when you become aware of all vehicles around you.

It helps greatly to turn your head to do a "shoulder check" to see if a car is in your blind spot that you cannot see with your mirrors. This is another one of those practices that you will never regret incorporating into your driving routine. There will be many more times than you would believe when you do see a car in your blind spot and avoid causing either of you to wreck. Also be aware if you are in another driver's blind spot. Either speed up or drop back or change lanes so that you do not contribute to an accident even if it is the driver's responsibility to watch out for you. Being in the "right" does nothing for you if you are injured. DuPont considered it an avoidable accident if we were the driver in someone else's blind spot and were involved in an accident. You were rewarded handsomely if you had a safe driver record, but if you had too many accidents, you would no longer be allowed to work where you would be using a company vehicle.

A huge safety lesson is to delay pulling into an intersection until someone else has "cleared" the intersection if there are other cars waiting also because of the danger of someone else not being able to stop prior to the intersection. Certainly always look left, right, left because the greater danger to the driver is from the left if in the U.S. In other countries you may need to look right, left, and right before entering the intersection.

A new mother with a child in the car is often the very safest driver on the road. They will hardly pull out if they can even see another car coming. We need to realize that not only are we worthy of avoiding an accident, but any passengers are also, and if you are the driver, then you are responsible for them also. That is really a frightening responsibility! As a part of our safe driving training we are encouraged to always drive even someone else's car because of our extensive driver training. I find very few drivers I am comfortable riding with, and that may be because I seldom ride with someone else driving. It is also a major problem that will definitely increase your stress just to be in an accident even if there is no injury involved. The paperwork, phone calls, estimates for repair, maybe a rental car (picking up and delivery), loss of value of your automobile, and the list goes on and on, even if there is not a legal aspect to deal with. Those legal aspects can certainly increase your stress level right over the top!

Road rage is a very real situation today, so we must absolutely not do <u>anything</u> to bring that situation on. The aggressor usually is not really angry at you, but their anger at something else is directed at you because they don't know you, probably won't see you again, and they are behind the wheel of an "instrument of destruction" if they choose to use it that way. I no longer allow anyone to tailgate me, if possible, but I also do not tap my brakes. I find a place to pull over safely and allow them to pass. I never flash my lights at anyone because they are not going the speed I desire, but I used to do that. If you watch your mirror adequately you can even anticipate other aggressive drivers and just give them even more room. These aggressive drivers will eventually cause an accident, but there is no reason you need to be the one to teach them a lesson.

Cruise control is another technological advance that can lower your stress level if you use it properly. It can reduce your concern about a speeding ticket while better allowing you to stay close to the speed you desire. It can also reduce your fatigue level, which may come about because you are not so worried about a speeding ticket and the negative impact it may have on your insurance premiums.

If you take time to focus on safety in all that you do, you will find that it is a wonderful investment in your peace level. Small changes, like having your clothing and valuables readily available in case of fire or any other emergency so you can dress quickly and take your valuables with you. If you have a fire, often the fire department or insurance or apartment owners will not allow you to go back to retrieve any items for weeks, months, maybe never. Keep a light (preferably a lamp that can be put on your head so you can have your hands free) near your head when sleeping. If the smoke alarm goes off, then roll out of the bed and put the light on to see if the smoke level is low in your room. If you stand up into the smoke, it may burn your eyes so badly that they will not open. Or if they do, they will be so filled with tears to wash out the smoke particles you will not be able to see. If you are already on the floor, you can crawl to an escape exit. Always have every family member and guest aware of the meeting place everyone is to go to in the event of a fire. The mailbox is what we use as a meeting point. Every bed has a light under it, and all smoke alarms are routinely verified.

Hire Backup for Computer

Few happenings are worse than having your computer crash! It is a definite stress reducer to have a service that backs up your computer off-site. Certainly there is a concern about security, but they address that adequately enough for me. The security I gain of not losing my data is far greater than the security I might lose by allowing someone else to know what is on my computer.

Comedy/Laughter—Increases Alpha-Endorphins

Laughter is wonderful for reducing stress! So often today, our laughter is at someone else's expense, and that will damage your relationship with others. So the overall outcome is negative. Some of the old shows on YouTube are wonderful sources of laughter. If you want an unlimited source of humor, just look at yourself and your actions (as I do so often). You will NEVER run out of material! If you focus on seeing the humor in situations, it will diminish the negativity of the awful happening. If you don't laugh at other's misfortunes, they may stop laughing at yours. If someone always is doing something to make you look bad, and reminds you of your mistakes often, or even has a nickname for you that has a negative connotation, then find a different friend. This is a "caustic" relationship. None of us needs that, and we certainly don't deserve it. Find someone who is more positive or be alone, because being alone is better than a negative relationship. There are some people who improve your life in either of two ways. One is to come into your life and the other is to leave it. Your health and future depend strongly on what stresses you, and if it is a person, then first attempt to rectify, then make several more attempts to rectify, because this person must have been important in your life at some time. If you have made enough attempts that you are satisfied you have done more than your part to change it into a positive relationship, then find someone who can make you laugh more.

Joke Books

Seldom do we see books that are primarily full of jokes, but often they are a part of other reading that you do. If a joke makes you laugh, then that is a true blessing! If they only amuse you, then they are still a blessing. Seek out something that makes you laugh when you can, and don't forget that you are often your best source of humor!

I started doing something that amuses me often and makes me smile. It is a way of making fun of myself and the situations I get into. I started it a few years ago about my wonderful neighbor who allows me to keep my horse on his farm for free. He and his wife are two of the happiest people I know, and they make me laugh every time I am around them. They see so much humor in life. Since Dick allows me to keep my horse on his property (which is just over the fence from my yard), I do some work up at his barn. His barn is full of so much stuff that we call it "Dick's museum." My granddaughter loves to explore it to see what all is in his museum.

Dick is a very successful businessman and was the very first Century 21 Real Estate office in Knoxville, Tennessee because they did not have everything in place when Dick signed on. Some of the stuff is from his business and homes he has acquired over the years; some items his children want him to store for them, and some are from many yard sale trips. Some of it is even worth something! He also has two horses, so I help him with them when I am cleaning up and feeding my horse. Since he is so very funny, I started what I have begun to call "Humorous Muttering." Stay with me now, I actually have not lost it. I just complain about how I have to do all the work (which is not true) and that he does not appreciate it (which he does) and that amuses me. He had a very old, almost worthless broom that I would sometimes use to sweep up the hall of the barn (or what you could see in between everything), so after telling him that he should at least get me a new one since I do all the work, I now just complain (to myself) not only do I have to work, work, work, but he won't even buy me a good broom! He makes me laugh all the time, even when he does not know it.

I use this also with my granddaughter because she uses my bathroom most of the time. I have a mirror so I can see to put my contacts in that she uses to put her makeup on. So, my humorous muttering with her is like, "I buy her books and send her to school, and she still uses my bathroom." This exercise only works if you are amused by it, as I am. I love having my granddaughter close in "my space," so I get some amusement from saying and thinking the things I do to bring me pleasure. She loves using my computer in my bedroom office even though she has her own excellent computer. She has even asked if she can have my room if I die, so that is now a running joke with us. She loves to sit in the chair when I am working on my computer, and when she was small enough, she loved to sit on my head and/or shoulders. So I often use the technique of humorous muttering where she can hear me. It includes "You have your own computer; why do you come in and attempt to take over my office."

If you do decide to use this technique of humorous muttering, be careful. Someone observing you might think you have been taking something or need to be taking something along with immediate hospitalization!

Limit Immediate Access to Yourself (You Are Not That Important)

One of the most stressful parts of our lives now is that just about anyone has access to us 24/7, or at least we think they should. We think we need to be accessible all the time. If you want to seriously reduce your stress level, then limit access to yourself at least part of the day and/or night. Few of us are so critical to the world that we must be on call 24/7. If you are that important, then take a break often and allow someone else to take over because if your stress makes you ill or you can't perform well in your tasks, then they will be taking over anyway. If you are that important, you need to have several others available to take over such important work. If the task is that important, it deserves several others to assist with it. And if they (whoever they are) feel you are that important, they should realize that everyone needs some downtime.

Really, it is okay *not* to be accessible some of the time. Often we burden ourselves because we want to know all that is going on even if we are taking some time away from the constant pressure. If you are informed of a problem but it is not your responsibility to assist in taking care of it, that puts you in the center of the action anyway and increases your stress level. A few times in my career I thought that what I was doing was important, but I soon realized that anything I could do someone else could do better, faster, with better quality, and for less money. Often our management team tells us we are that important because it takes a burden off of them if you are willing to be available 24/7.

I turn my phone off often and have as yet to be in a situation where it was absolutely necessary that I was available. Maybe my job is not as important as your job, but if it causes you more stress than mine does, you should be begging for help and looking for some relief!

Money

Money, whether you have a great deal or little money, is a great stressor! I don't have enough space to deal with this subject except to ask you to read, attend classes, or seek professional help to deal with this subject if it is a problem for you. Money can ruin many a friendship, marriage, or close relationship quickly, and for life. Just like the suggestions we have discussed about water, proper food, and adequate rest are so simple, so is money. Don't spend more than you can afford! Now that is so easy to say, but today financial institutions keep throwing opportunities at us to spend their money so they can make those exorbitant interest rates. I remember one time when my money was especially tight and my car needed almost two thousand dollars' work on the transmission. I asked if this national transmission shop had a payment plan. They said they did, so I authorized the repair. When I went back to pick up the car, I was told I had to go to the office of the finance company. The interest rate was 32%! I went to my local bank for a signature loan at a much lower interest rate to retrieve my car. I was appalled that many people have to pay this exorbitant interest, but they must because the company is still in business.

One thing that will help reduce your stress with money is to refrain from buying a new car unless you have all or at least most of the money to pay for it. The first few months the payments seem like nothing because you have your dream wheels and you think you don't have to pay for the service in the beginning, but you do! All new cars have a part of the total price an average of what it costs the manufacturer to keep them going. The dealer you take them to for repair during the warranty also makes money because they send the bill to the manufacturer. The manufacturer allows the dealer to make enough money to be willing to work on their cars without question to keep the customer feeling good about their purchase. When you are into the later years of the payment that seemed so small at your first purchase time, it now seems like you are responsible for the national debt. Plus the media attempts to convince you that your car is almost obsolete and it is time to trade again. If you think you are "stealing" the car from the dealer, you are almost if not totally delusional. They make their money or they do not sell or stay in business for very long. You might use this same method on any large purchase that you have to finance except your home.

Increase Rewards to Yourself

Here is another area where you need to be a little selfish or look out for yourself if you are not already. No one is going to be as good to you as you can be to yourself in most cases. Only you know what would please you, so at least plan to achieve that goal no matter how long it takes (and if it does not harm someone else or a special relationship). We deserve to be good to ourselves some of the time but certainly not all of the time. Many are stressed because they are attempting to take care of everyone else and not themselves. This goes back to the just saying NO concept as well as saying YES to yourself...sometimes and within reason.

Large Rewards

We need to plan some large rewards for ourselves and those who are important to us. A large reward may be a vacation or anything that is attainable and wise. Often we think we need a bigger house, but we don't, so maybe we need to drop that off the list. A large reward is very stress releasing because it is something we can plan toward, something we desire, and the journey is often very calming because we know we are making progress toward our goal.

Small Rewards

A small reward may be a walk at lunch to allow us to decompress from a morning of hard, productive work. Even that small reward can be refreshing because we most often enjoy a walk outside, and it is a reward for focusing for several hours. A movie or a special meal or some item of clothing can be an excellent reward if it is in "payment" for your hard work. If it is just because you wanted it, the activity or purchase does not seem as justified.

Vacations

Vacations are *critical* to reducing stress, but even they can be stressful as evidenced by the Holmes and Rahe scale, counting for thirteen points. The best way to have an enjoyable vacation is to plan for it months in advance and even pay for it if you can prior to going. A planned vacation is usually a better vacation than a spontaneous one, but the greatest benefit is the anticipation of the good, restful time you are going to have in a few months.

When you have a well-planned, restful vacation, the long-term benefits can last for several months because now you have a very pleasant time to look back upon with delight. This long-term anticipation *and* reflection afterward can give you tangible benefits for up to a year.

Spontaneous vacations are also restful, but they do not have the anticipation factor and may not have the reflection benefit because the anticipation was not as great. So a good combination of both is very useful, but the one with the longer planning is more stress reducing.

Do whatever you can to take a two-week vacation even if part of the time is getting ready to go, vacation time for a week, and then a few days to get ready to go back to the other world. I remember the first time I told my family that we were going on a two-week vacation. They asked how I could do that because they knew some about my work—for most of my career I have worked from my home office. I told them it was easy. If anything came up that was not important, it could wait until I returned. If something came up that was really important, my boss would have to be informed, so I may as well let him/her take care of it in my absence. In all the years nothing (about work) kept me from taking this vacation.

Vacations are to reduce your stress, but often they don't because we don't go on vacation. We take our work with us! And we can do that so much easier now with our new "work anywhere" technology.

I cannot emphasis this enough: When you are on vacation, *be* on vacation! If you check your email, voice mail, snail mail, or any other communication even for a few minutes, you may as well be at work for the *entire* day. Don't ever, ever call the office to see how things are going! If you do, you should just count that as an office day; even if there is nothing you need to see about, you have already prepared your mind to work even if for just a few minutes. Not only that, but most of those back at the office don't want to hear about your good time, and they may even be glad you are gone! Don't do this to yourself or your family. It will ruin your vacation and actually increase your stress; you know you need and deserve a break, but YOU have made the decision to attempt to work when you should not be.

This is also very difficult on your family if you work when they are with you. Small children want your attention all the time because you are the most important person in their lives right now. This is also an excellent time to catch up with older children and maybe even your spouse, when you can focus on family rather than spend some time working. I assure you, you will regret not taking a full vacation of relaxation time to de-stress. Be good to yourself and relax as much as possible.

Spiritual

I have not discussed spiritual aspects regarding stress because I know many (and sometimes most) don't want to hear about that part. If you don't have a spiritual part of your life, then I would encourage you to seek knowledge of what that can do for you in reducing stress.

If you do have a spiritual part of your life and it is not reducing your stress level, then find one that does. The spiritual part should bring you some peace and stress relief. This is a big part of my life and it helps me greatly when I am dealing with overwhelming stress (like at this time of my life). My stress numbers are so high, it would be very scary except for the offset of my spiritual life. I would hope you have the same.

Contact Friends

Contacting old friends can do a great deal to reduce your stress. Sometimes just listening to their voice on their answering service is pleasant. These are the kind of friends where, even if it has been years since you saw them, it seems like it was just yesterday. This is a very real advantage of social media, and I enjoy keeping up with so many others this way. The disadvantage of using social media only is that others do not often tell you their difficulties and troubles, so you may think you are the only one with problems and the rest of the world is happy!

Be "Real"

One concept that my father instilled in me from early childhood that has allowed me to deal with stress (especially when the stress is caused by others) is to realize that I am no better than anyone on this entire earth, no matter their station in life or what has happened to them. My parents were always giving and helping other families in any way they could. This greatly helped me realize how blessed I was as a child.

I know this deep understanding that I am not better than anyone else has served me very well as I spent the last several years giving medically underserved patients the very best care I could. One of my very first patients was complaining of serious abdominal pain, and it was obvious that he had a large hernia that could only be corrected by surgery. He even had health insurance but had suffered with this for six years and could not find anyone who would help him. I was absolutely appalled that he had gone this long without appropriate care when he had insurance that would cover the surgical costs! All it took from me was one simple sheet of paper on my clinic letterhead with his name, symptoms of abdominal pain (I did not even have to know the diagnosis), and two words, "surgical referral," along with my signature. He went to the surgeon we referred him to, had the surgery, found that he actually had two hernias (one much larger than the other), and recovered without any lingering pain after the surgical pain was over. He was so very grateful and talks about it practically every time I see him. I was angry with our current healthcare system that this man suffered for over six years, had adequate insurance, but could not get proper care! How many others need something as simple as a few words on a sheet of paper to bring them medical relief?

Many of my patients complain that even if they do have insurance, they are treated poorly by other providers because their insurance is government funded. Most say the provider never even looks at them or even touches them but just keeps their attention on the paperwork and then gives them a prescription and moves on quickly, leaving the impression that the patient is not worth their time. It was amazing to hear these stories so often by so many credible people who were not chronic complainers. It was also amazing to me how appreciative these patients were if you treated them with dignity. They were not accustomed to being treated as an equal (which is what they deserve), and it endeared them to our clinic. They felt appreciated. My upbringing of never looking down on anyone has helped me so many times in improving my relationships with others. It has allowed me to have many new friends and patients who appreciate all of us at the clinics. So, if you have good insurance and access to proper healthcare then your stress should be a great deal less than those that do not.

Unfortunately, we often encounter others who think they are better than we are. That is tragic on their part. This attitude leads to arrogance. People who are arrogant or feel that they are better than others are usually persons of low self-esteem, which is what makes this difficult for them. Often they fear that others might think them "ordinary" and not really special, so their actions are almost demanding of acceptance. It really is wonderful and stress relieving just being ordinary. When you gain success in being recognized as someone of special status, it is often very short-lived and can cause others to search diligently into you and your past to bring you back down to earth or at least to ordinary status again. One attitude that has helped me *tremendously* is to consider everyone I meet to be smarter than I am. The good thing about this attitude is that I am seldom wrong! I learn something useful from each and every person I meet, and I am constantly amazed how much other people know.

We need to self-evaluate to have a better life that is less stressful. It is very difficult and certainly stressful to continue to keep up the façade of being someone who is better than others. No one likes to be disrespected, but there were times in my life when I was an abject fool. It is shameful to say that about myself, but when I look back on some of my mistakes, I can't believe I acted the way I did. Some of my mistakes were just within the realm of human error, but some were where I made a conscious decision that was certainly the WRONG decision.

We are each and every one unique in this world, and some appear more unique than others! I have found that I have been wrong about others, and after overcoming my own weakness and getting to know that person, they had a great deal to offer. We need to understand that we are different and important to this world, but we should also realize that we are not too important. I am often reminded of this when I fly. I tell myself, "If you were so important, then people on the ground would just be waiting for your plane to pass over them." That thought helps keep me in perspective. I am not important in this world, but I am as important as anyone else.

There are so many people who have achieved great success, and I am pleased to know about them and even personally know a few of these blessed folks. I too have had a blessed life without drawing too much attention to myself, and I am very content with that. I even struggle with being recognized when I have not had a one-on-one chance to meet another person who may have attended a seminar I presented somewhere. I am somewhat embarrassed that someone has the advantage of knowing my name when I have not had the privilege of knowing theirs personally.

One of the ways of opening any conversation with someone

I am not absolutely certain knows my name is to say, "My name is Gary Bickford and it is good to see you." Often the person says, "Oh, I know your name" out of kindness to me when they really did have my name associated with my face. This is essential to having a good conversation—it is so embarrassing and detrimental to good conversation to not listen to what the person is saying because your brain is busy attempting to remember their name.

This is why anyone who is in marketing wears an easily read name tag to identify them and their company, just so the person will be able to listen to everything you are saying rather than searching for your name in their name and face data bank. It is "good business" as well as a courtesy to others to assist them with your name, face, and affiliation so you can have a good conversation from the very beginning. There has been much research conducted to justify the expense of appropriate name tags. I keep a supply of the temporary name tags at home so that anytime I entertain, everyone finds it easier to interact with each other by everyone (even me) wearing a name tag. It is just good entertaining etiquette.

Another stress reducer to any conversation is never to be offended if someone does not remember your name. If that offends you, then it might be time to evaluate your importance in this world and be somewhat thankful that not everyone knows who you are. Any of us are subject to being with someone we want to introduce, but for some reason we can't remember their name! This is so embarrassing to everyone, so I often tell the person with me to just introduce themselves if they are comfortable with that. As we age, our contacts data base has grown quite large, and it may take our brain a few seconds to "search" even if we recognize a face. Our brains were the first computer to use face recognition software or "brain ware." I worked with a woman in the clinical business, and she seemed to be impressed with how many people I knew, so I asked how old she was. After she told me, I informed her that I was twenty years older than she was and therefore had two decades of opportunity of knowing people that she had not had time to meet yet. I probably should not have told her that because I don't think she was impressed with me after she realized I was just "ordinary."

Please keep in mind the difficulty of your name if you are saddled with a name that is difficult to understand and pronounce, as mine is. I have had so much difficulty with people mispronouncing my name that when I make reservations at a restaurant I don't use my real name. I started out using the name "Jones" until one time a real Jones signed up right after me. I explained this situation to our small dinner party, and one of them suggested that I just use the name Ford. So I have used that name for reservations for places where your real name does not matter and does not require identification. That has worked well for me except for one time several years ago when one of my best friends and also a big customer was driving his family into town to meet my family at a restaurant. They had some minor car trouble and called the restaurant to pass the message along to me, but since I was registered under Ford rather than my full name, we were not able to get together that evening. When I tell others about this, they think it is humorous, especially when the hostess appears to be about fourteen years old and mispronounces your name to everyone who is waiting to be seated. I often ask these young ladies, "Does your mother know you are pretending to be working as an adult?"

Each of us is important, but it is somewhat "attitude adjusting" when we realize that the world goes on without us, even when we think we are set up for something special, like to present a seminar. One time I was flying into a small town to present a seminar and ran into a friend from some years back. We were talking about our history together, and I purposely waited to be the last one to board so we could extend the visit since he was telling me about his wife and children. Just as the last three of us passengers were at the gate

BE "REAL"

to have our ticket scanned, they announced that the plane was now at its maximum loading capacity and no one else could board. That was potentially very stressful—I knew that my company had scheduled me to give this seminar, and several people had signed up because they received continuing education credits (CEU) to keep their medical certification current.

The airline gave each of the three of us free tickets to fly anywhere in the U.S. I already had many frequent flyer miles in that airline's account, so I decided a way for me and my company to look good in this was to have a drawing for this free ticket among those who came to the seminar. The person who won the ticket called the next day to express their gratitude because now they could go to the national convention in addition to this regional meeting. I believe the national convention was in San Francisco that year, and I hoped to see them there because that is one of my favorite places to visit. Sometime later I asked the organizer of the meeting that I missed how the meeting went, and he said it was a great meeting, so I knew I was not really missed. Actually, almost immediately he remembered that I had not been able to come so he said, "Of course, it would have been better if you had been there," but I knew at least the one person who received the free ticket was glad I was not able to make it.

Realizing you are really not that important can also help reduce your feelings of paranoia (the feeling that someone is out to get you). I have had a few patients who were under another provider for their paranoia, and the problem was well controlled with their current medication. They would always tell me that it took several drug changes to achieve a satisfactory result. The even fewer patients I was able to diagnose with paranoia I never attempted to treat because I was not qualified and not familiar with the multiple drugs or how to appropriately manage them to help the patient. I felt so helpless to assist my patients with paranoia because I was not able to "reason" with them enough to show that their feelings might be unfounded. Several felt that every word they said was being recorded as well as every action, which was similar to the negative situations of very famous individuals. I attempted to point out that they were very important to me and their family, but in reality they were not important enough for someone to monitor them 24/7. They always had a reason why and nebulous data to prove their point. When I asked who might be after them, there was never a solid answer but always "they." This situation is very stressful for the patient and for all their acquaintances and family. A few patients were obviously suffering from paranoia, but would not allow me to refer them to someone who was qualified to help them, nor were they willing to seek a specialist on their own. This constant concern that someone is after you is often why criminals turn themselves in to law enforcement—they have such a poor life due to the constant vigilance they must continue. This is one of the reasons why wealthy people often have such big homes, with all different types of entertainment available, because they cannot be comfortable out in the general public. For people who are not wealthy enough to have their own hideaway, the pressure is even greater because they have to be in the public domain all the time. I grieve for the patients I was not able to convince to seek proper treatment for this condition. It helps us all to realize that we are not really that important. I hope to always be that way. I want to help others and am willing to deal with any "recognition" negatives if I ever get to that level if it allows me to help others. I certainly don't want it for myself, ever.

Take Naps or Refreshing Breaks

Research has shown—and common sense substantiates—that you are more productive if you focus on work for a time and then take a refreshing break than if you attempt to work without appropriate breaks. I often encourage others to set an alarm to work for so long and then if need be also set the alarm on how long to break. Unfortunately breaks are often more fun than work, even if you work for yourself.

I am so very blessed with the ability to take quick "power naps" and awaken quickly also, but I know of many others who cannot do that. They feel worse if they take a nap and are less productive. If that is true in your case, then find another way to make your breaks refreshing.

My quick naps allow me to go to sleep right away, and after about twenty minutes or so I awaken on my own. This has allowed me to accomplish a great deal when I work at a place conducive to a quick nap. I learned to do this as a teenager when I would go home for lunch and be able to nap during that time and still make it back to work within the hour. All the years that I traveled, I learned to nap in my company car. I honestly believe I could almost be asleep by the time the seat was fully reclined. When I awakened I did not have to get out of the car to walk around or throw cold water in my face. I could just awaken, raise the seat back up, and start driving.

One time this did cause me a real problem. I was having a more difficult time staying awake, so I pulled way to the back of a truck stop and fell asleep quickly. I had parked where there were no trucks near me because they might think I was ill or dead, and I didn't want to concern anyone else. During my nap a truck pulled up in front of my car where I was facing the trailer as if I would be driving under it. While sleeping I was dreaming I was still driving and that a truck had jackknifed (where the trailer starts coming around faster than the tractor is pulling it), and I had recognized the danger, but the trailer was coming toward me faster than I could stop. I awoke as we often do in "terror dreams" so glad that it was a dream and not reality. Well, the first thing I saw was the trailer that had parked in front of me so closely that the entire windshield was showing only the side of the trailer! So, I awakened from a terror dream to have all my senses think that it was real! I almost broke the brake pedal because my body was reacting from a full adrenaline-fueled panic! It took me several seconds to realize the car was not moving and that the truck (and my car) were actually parked. Needless to say, I was not sleepy for several hours after that too realistic, terror-filled awakening. Talk about immense stress condensed into a micro-second of time!

Exercise is another refreshing break to keep your productivity high. It is not always easy to exercise at work due to time restraints and the need to worry about perspiration on your work clothes. If you work in a building that has stairs, an excellent, refreshing break is to walk the stairs. I have used this for years because walking the stairs is certainly a good exercise to increase blood flow! The good thing about this exercise is that you don't have to change clothing, it is within your building, and you are not observed because many people avoid the stairs unless there is an emergency. You can take your time and climb at your own pace, stop when you need to, and return to your work refreshed. You can also feel good intellectually because you have been able to exercise some during the day. If you were to do this three or four times a day, it could be as beneficial as walking a mile or so when you get home. Climbing the stairs is

TAKE NAPS OR REFRESHING BREAKS

somewhat different than walking or running, so you may feel some slight tenderness in your calf muscles when you first begin. I remember one time when I was in Puerto Rico and it was raining too hard to run one morning, so I spent the same amount of time climbing stairs as I usually did running. That was a mistake! I could walk normally only if I overcame the pain in the muscles in my lower leg. I was amused about the pain because I had never realized the difference in running or walking and climbing stairs. It still is a great exercise, but I have learned to do it in moderation.

A different break for you may be to read a book for a change from your work. This only works for me if I can discipline myself to only read for the reasonable break time rather than reading the rest of the book. When I have a big project to do (like writing this book) I know that I cannot even *start* a book because it will definitely interfere with my work focus even when I attempt to convince myself that reading someone else's work might benefit my writing.

Another break idea may be to visit with someone who takes the break at the same time, but if you talk about business, it could turn into a negative break. Any break should be refreshing for you, if possible. It may even be a call home as long as it is a positive call most of the time. For some, calling home is just a report on the negative things that are happening. I know of some who have to ask, "Well, did anything positive happen to the kids today?"

A break from a task is always a good idea, if it's possible for you to take one. You may have to put some thought into what type of activity would cause your breaks to be of more benefit. It may take you some time to attempt different activities to help, but it is a good investment in yourself to do so. Also, you might encourage others who are important in your life to take breaks whenever possible. I encourage all mothers to rest when their little "charges" are resting rather than working because children take so much energy to just keep them safe when they are awake. If you have had children, you will most certainly believe that children do truly have a guardian angel looking after them no matter how diligent you are about their safety. Some of our children need a whole team of guardian angels due to their physical aggressiveness even if they are female. I know that with my two daughters and now my granddaughter, I have had what I thought was hyper-vigilance about their safety, but they still needed that angel at times!

Music

Music is a wonderful stress reducer. Many businesses invest a good deal of money selecting music that calms you in areas you need to be calmer and can also be targeted to cause you to purchase certain items. If the business is entertainment, the most popular music is designed to excite you rather than calm you. Sometimes the calm after the excitement of the more stimulating music is better than if you had not experienced the stirring music that refreshed your spirit.

If you go to sleep with music that keeps playing, your brain will hear the music even if you are asleep. This ability is a self-defense and natural protection so you can hear a threat or disturbance, but it can also work against you if your brain listens to music that is designed to increase excitement when your brain and body need restorative rest. I have often been in places where there is more than one type of music playing at the same time, and my poor little brain just can't deal with that much stimulation at one time. Maybe yours can.

I most often drive without listening to any music unless I begin to tire and feel that listening to some exciting music will keep me awake, as it often does. I have a very good friend who is one of the smartest men I know, and it seems that he knows everything about good music. He came to the southwest U.S. to join me on a five-day ATV riding adventure in Arizona and Utah. I was already in the area because I was working for ten weeks as a senior family nurse practitioner student in Monument Valley, Utah, in a clinic that serves the

Navajo population. Since I had driven out, I had my own vehicle, so I picked him up at the airport and we spent five wonderful days exploring that beautiful part of the world. I never turned on my radio while we were driving for many hours because everything out there is a long ways from anywhere else! He is a very kind and courteous person to others, so he never even asked if we could listen to the radio. Later after we were both back at home in Tennessee, he remarked on that fact, and I was so embarrassed that I did not realize that music was such a big part of his life. Actually, on the Navajo reservation (which is the largest Nation of Native Americans), most of the local stations use the native language, and it was so interesting to hear their beautiful language for a few seconds; then an American word would slip in, like "Wal-Mart." After my good friend expressed disbelief that I could go for five days without listening to the radio, he was really blown away when I told him I drove the 1,900-plus-mile trip without turning it on either going or returning home. I must have a brain that needs to think quietly and is not capable of thinking deeply and listening to stimulating music at the same time.

Please realize the value of taking a break from a focused task. Then put something into place that is good enough to cause you to look forward to your next break and also allows you to be more refreshed and productive when you get back on task.

Forgive

I imagine some of you are thinking that this is a "spiritual" chapter, but are you aware that big corporations have training classes that include *forgiveness*? The main reason is that this money spent is "good for business!" Can you believe that? Actually, I am certain that those who focus on the spiritual part of their life would be surprised to hear that it is not only a spiritual attribute but is valued in business! Even PTSD can be greatly reduced by forgiving.

How in the world can forgiveness be good for business? The answer is simple enough to convince upper management to spend the money and time that employees would not be doing their regular job to be able to attend a training session. When you are in the business world, every time you take an employee away from their assigned task, you had better have an excellent reason because they were hired (and are paid) to do a specific task or responsibility. Education is a very important part of any business, but each and every hour of training must be justified and authorized by upper management. This justification really comes evident when you own your own business and it means money out of your pocket to conduct any training session.

So the fact that businesses conduct training sessions that include forgiveness is a *very* significant occurrence in the business world. It is also expensive because you usually hire a professional training person or group or have your own training group, which may be even more expensive. You have the trainer's fee, travel expenses, training material expense, food, and certainly the expense of taking the attendees away from their designated work responsibilities.

Forgiveness is _good for **you**_! Be selfish at times in your search to reduce or handle your stress better, to improve your lifestyle and possibly extend your life while increasing your quality of life. Do you know who the most selfish person is in the entire world? The answer may surprise you: a newborn baby! If you have had a child, you will now be nodding your head yes, and if you have not had children yet, you will remember this statement (not because I have given some great revelation but because it is universally true). Have you ever tried to reason with a newborn who is crying? If so, you are wasting your time. You should be calling 911, or HELP, or getting some food or changing a diaper (if you can't get someone else to do it for you). When a baby is crying they don't care where they are or where you are or what you are doing, no matter how important it is to you or even the entire universe! You can ask them to delay, wait, stop, go away, or anything else you can think of, but NOTHING works but to satisfy their immediate needs. You can even have the following conversation with them: "If you stop crying for five minutes, I will buy you either a new Mercedes-Benz sports car or a Lear jet when you turn sixteen; actually, I will give you _both_ a new car and a new jet if you will stop crying for ten minutes right now." It is not going to work; truly nothing is going to work! Thank goodness those newborn babies sleep most of the twenty-four hours in a day, because even the best of parents cannot deal with that extreme selfishness.

Thankfully our parents dealt with this period of our life when we were the _definition_ of selfishness and then spent the rest of our childhood teaching us _not_ to be selfish at least most of the time. Our not being selfish is a learned attribute that some learn better than others. This attribute works very well in much of our lives, and it is very desirable in ourselves and others around us.

So, I want you to realize that some selfishness is good for dealing with stress in your life. Forgive others for *yourself*, not for others. This may seem like a bizarre concept, but just remember that if the business world thinks it is valuable enough to spend a good deal of money and resources on teaching forgiveness, then it is important for you to at least strongly consider it—even if it goes against your wonderful, lifelong training of not being selfish.

Remember, this is not necessarily a spiritual benefit *only*, but is also really good for *YOU*. You are the only one really in control of how you deal with stress. Others may help you with stress or cause you more stress, but you are the only one who really deals with it. Advice is only good if you take it, and often advice is invaluable! You should forgive because it relieves you of a great deal of stress that never becomes less but only becomes worse if you do not forgive. If you (I have to work on this greatly) have someone you need to forgive, it is therapeutic to do so! The sooner the better.

Forgiving someone else may be one of the most difficult personal tasks you ever perform in your entire life! But, forgiveness is so necessary to benefit your overall life, work, personal relationships, and certainly your spiritual life. One of the difficulties of forgiveness is that you have to remember the reason why you need to forgive another, and the process brings up the reason again, which can be difficult and sometimes devastating if you have suppressed that memory for some time. This is similar to when a judge tells a jury to disregard a statement because the jury has to remember the statement in order to forget it; they have to repeat the statement in their mind to begin the process of disregarding it because we do not have the capability of totally forgetting. The lawyer who made the statement may want the judge to say "disregard this statement" because it works for them—the jury hears the statement orally and other times in their thoughts and thereby imprints it deeper into their memory.

Please remember that forgiving others is best for you, and you really must forgive *everyone*. Now this is where the maturity you have has to demonstrate itself. Certainly some are easier to forgive than others, and it is really difficult to forgive *everyone*.

Let's start with the easier ones first because we need success early in this difficult journey or we will not "stay the course." The benefit to industry and business when you forgive others is that it removes that negative process of remembering the need to forgive and allows the employee to be more productive and therefore more valuable to the "bottom line" of helping the business be successful.

The others at your work certainly need to be on the list because we spend so many hours and such a large part of our life at work. This is a good place to start because we very often have others at work who have done something real or imagined that have caused us grief. Most often it is a supervisor who has either done something to us or not done something for us that we wanted them to do. I do not want to mitigate or lessen your reason for having negative feelings about supervisors because I have been blessed to have good supervisors and also some of the very worst. I will say that as a manager and owner of several clinics, the responsibility of supervising others is the most difficult part of your working career! Even people who are better at managing others than I am agree that it is the most difficult task of all. You can take every educational opportunity to learn to be a good manager, and those opportunities can be of great benefit, but they still don't adequately prepare you for supervising others.

Oftentimes we become angry with someone who is supervising us when they were just doing their job, and actually doing it well. Seldom do we enjoy telling someone else what to do, and some deal with this far better than others, but I doubt that anyone enjoys having someone else instruct them on how to do things differently, even if we easily recognize the need to change. I have had employees make the statement, "It was the way they said it!" if they know they were incorrect and had no justifiable defense for what they needed to change. There really is no way to sugar-coat a criticism from a supervisor at work. Certainly supervisors are trained to say positive things first, and some of them actually do that, but nearly all of that is forgotten when the conversation gets around to the negative side of something we should have done differently. This situation is similar to saying, "You look ugly" and then attempting to convince the person that you were only kidding. That will never happen because the other person only heard "ugly," and that is such a damaging word to our psyche that it cannot be undone no matter how much you recant your words. Another similar situation is when a person is told that they have cancer. Most stop listening and start planning their death details, no matter how mild a cancer is or what the survival rate may be or how successful the treatment is. That is why it is a good idea to take someone with you if you anticipate any serious discussions.

Early in my limited medical training, I read a book about a physician who had practiced for forty years in New York City as a family practice specialist. He had a very successful female patient in for a routine physical exam, including a breast exam, which he did with the patient both sitting and lying down. During his thorough examination, he felt what he thought was a lump in her breast while she was sitting up. He felt the same lump in the same place when she was lying down. He remarked in his excellent book (I apologize for not citing the reference to his book because it was years ago and I can't find the reference) that he knew when he told her he had determined that she had a lump in her breast, her life would be changed *forever*! He further related that this devastating news would be so damaging to her that he wanted it confirmed as soon as possible by further testing to determine if it was cancerous or not (benign). This was such an important lesson for me to learn and use in my work as a family nurse practitioner. I am not trained to ever diagnose anyone with cancer, so I always send them to a specialist as soon as possible.

I had a medical assistant who was to check the patient in, take their vital signs, and ask some of the beginning questions about the symptoms and/or purpose of their visit. A patient I had seen for some time who was usually upbeat in demeanor seemed not his usual self during my part of the visit. I asked him why he was not his usual positive self, and he asked if his recent laboratory tests indicated that he had cancer. I had already reviewed them, but I did so again in his presence and allowed him to view them with me as I commented on them. Then I asked him why he was worried (and he certainly showed external signs of extreme stress). He said the medical assistant who checked him in had said that his test could indicate cancer. Of course, cancer is always a possibility for any of us since every cell in our body is growing and is replaced on a documented schedule, and cancer is when they grow and reproduce too fast. But for her to even mention the word "cancer" was, and almost always is, devastating to this patient. It took me some time to convince him that she was absolutely wrong to tell him that, even if he did have cancer, and that none of the tests we had performed indicated anything but normal results. Needless to say we had to find someone to replace her right away.

The point of this discussion about cancer is to say that hearing something negative about yourself is devastating to most people. Even people who seem like they can handle anything don't want to hear negative things said about them, especially if this person is your supervisor. I can remember nearly every annual evaluation over my long career, and even if it was a good one it seems that I remembered the negative far longer and thought of it more often than the positive part.

Most supervisors learn quickly to focus on the positive early and spend more time there before getting to the part that "hurts," or they will be unhappy as a manager. Also, unfortunately, we seldom have meetings or time in the office of the supervisor unless there is a problem. I wish we could have more meetings and just say "thanks to all of you for doing the best job that you can under the circumstances and that we are not going to ask you to leave here with a task to complete for our next meeting." So almost any interaction you have with management has the potential of being negative. I had a clinic manager who kept saying "you're fired" in a joking way, so I called her in to tell her that if you have the authority to fire someone, then that statement is *never* funny, but it could possibly be used if you don't have the authority to fire anyone. Another employee would tell other employees "you are in trouble now" in my hearing when I asked someone to come to my office so we could talk. I purposely corrected her in front of the other staff (which is not usually a good idea, but I wanted everyone to hear what I had to say) and told her that they may be getting a raise or promotion, so I did want that statement used again. I could have just talked to her alone, but somehow I had to get the message to everyone, and I could not depend on her to tell everyone that she had made a mistake.

The bottom line here is that a part of our work is hearing some negative statements from our manager because they often have a real need to correct us; none of us is perfect (fortunately) and we all make mistakes. Also, they may be required to always say something negative so we could suggest some improvement in their review of our performance as I did when I managed others, even knowing that the negative part would be remembered most and could drive a wedge in our working relationship.

Start realizing what a difficult job it is to be a manager if you don't already have on-the-job training to drive that point home deep into your brain, and allow that thought to help you begin your process of forgiving any (and every) manager who has caused you grief. This is an excellent start on changing your life for you and not because someone else mandated this difficult exercise. I assure you, you will not ever regret forgiving others.

I remember reading a quote that was attributed to Betsy Ross (she had something to do with designing our American flag) that when she was reminded of an offense someone had done to her, her reply was, "I distinctly remember forgetting about that." We discussed earlier that you really can't forget some things in your life, but we need to choose to not remember if we are going to forgive our managers at work.

What do we do if they are no longer our manager or have moved on to another company or even died? <u>Forgive them!</u> It is amazing that we humans allow someone to affect us so much even if they are dead! But they certainly can if we don't become selfish and forgive them. One speaker I heard said he uses the technique of speaking to the "dead" person (probably best done while alone and unobserved) as if they are still alive and sitting across from you in a chair. He suggested that you don't rehash why you need to forgive them, but you say (out loud), "I forgive you for everything you did to me or everything you did not do for me!" I have not used the chair, but I have done the same technique for some of the horrible managers I have had in my career. It is like a catharsis (cleansing) to be able to do this even if the other person is not aware (by being dead) that you have gone through this process for yourself and not really involved them.

What if those who are living don't ask you to forgive them? First of all, that's not going to happen, and you might as well greatly lower your unrealistic expectations for that miracle to come about. Often others don't even know that they have given you reason to need to forgive them. Those who do know they have offended probably will not apologize because it shows that they are "human" and therefore less than perfect. So if you are going to wait until someone asks you to forgive them, even if they are still alive, it is best for *you* to just forgive them anyway.

What about getting with the person and telling them that you forgive them? Not a good idea! First, you will have to dredge up the offensive situation, which adds to your stress level, and secondly the other person may not even remember the offense and will express disappointment that you even felt the way you do. Also, if it was something negative, it could even get worse with the discussion about the incident. Historically we usually get more stressed or angry every time we retell the story or go over it in our mind, so we don't want to go there. It is somewhat like the adage that "We don't want to get even: we want to get ahead!" in the hurting someone else business, so a conversation is generally fruitless. You can avoid the stress by just **forgiving everyone for everything!**

Now that we have been successful forgiving those who have been in a managerial role over us, what about our peers? Or maybe they used to be our peers and now they have been promoted—what do we think about that? The only thing worse is to get promoted where now YOU are the manager over your peers! I had this happen to me one time in my career, and it was a disaster! Two of the employees under my position, who were more experienced than I was and had had a long career, were fired. I did not have the authority to fire them by myself as I have as the sole owner of my business. In order to fire someone at DuPont, several people have to agree because it is a very serious happening. One of the men who were fired later told me that it was a good thing because he was now happier than he had ever been. That was very kind of him to say because I had tremendous respect for him. In reality, my boss did the actual firing in my presence. My boss was one of those on my list of bosses that I had to forgive, and he was very close to the top of that list! When we called this employee in to tell him he was terminated, my boss had told me that we were going to spend a great deal of time telling him what an excellent employee he had been for many years. Now things had changed for him, so we were very concerned about his behavior, and that was what I was prepared to hear and make any comments, if warranted. We had only been meeting for a minute or so when my boss said, "You are fired!" I was devastated that we treated this valuable employee with such rudeness. So when you are promoted over your peers, your stress level may go through the roof.

Since we spend so much time with our work peers and even more so than we often spend with our manager, we have more opportunities for something to happen that can cause us to have negative feelings about this person. Sometimes they hurt us without even realizing it, so again in this situation you would be better served if you just forgave everything and do not even attempt to discuss it with them. There is little profit from resurrecting the past, but great profit from totally forgiving and making a concerted effort to forget as much as possible.

Sometimes I hear people say, "I have to forgive myself before I can forgive others." Actually, I feel this could be a cop-out, an excuse for not moving forward in the effort to forgive others. This position is often viewed as "humble," a person who is so concerned about what they have done to others that they cannot even begin to think of forgiving others.

You are much better off if you start with others, for two main reasons. The first reason is that it is easier to forgive others than ourselves. Consider taking the easier way first, so again you can have a successful track record and that will make it easier for you to go to the next level. Forgiving others cannot be done until you realize that they are human and subject to mistakes in all parts of their life, even dealing with a person who is as perfect and wonderful as you are! We all make mistakes and one of the beauties of not being media fodder is that not many people know about them. Unfortunately, someone, somewhere, will find out about your mistakes and feel an overwhelming responsibility to remind you of them and broadcast them as widely as possible.

The second reason it is better to forgive others before forgiving yourself is that when you focus on forgiving others, it reminds you that you also are human. Therefore your mistakes are more easily understood and forgiven, and you can begin to live with yourself. We have all made mistakes that we regret deeply in all areas of our lives (at least I know I have), and for our own selfish reasons we need to move on past them. Hanging on to our own mistakes is actually worse than keeping a "running tab" on the mistakes others have made that caused us discomfort. This is because we know our mistakes, and others may know some of our mistakes, but they don't know *all* of our mistakes, thank goodness! Once you have convinced yourself of the value of forgiving others for your sake, then it will be easier to forgive yourself for your sake. It is humbling to know about our mistakes, and while we really can't forget them even if we wanted to, there is some value in remembering our mistakes. The value could be that it gives us the wherewithal not to make the same one again. Often we continue to make the same mistake over and over, and that is doubly troubling because we now know better the consequences of what we did before.

The good thing about forgiving yourself is that it can free your mind to know that you have forgiven others as well as yourself. You will be better able to recognize your mistakes and say "I am not perfect, of course, but I want to do the best I can." You can't be the best you can if you are still struggling with forgiving yourself because you have this albatross (bird of the sea that indicates bad luck) riding on your shoulder. This goes back to the idea that we are no better than anyone, and no one is better than we are because we all make mistakes. Some are just more visible than others, and we want to keep the ones that are not well known to others as discreetly quiet as we can. No one gains when we tell the things in our life that cause us shame or embarrassment.

It seems that some people don't ever forget anything negative about anyone, and often you know of the truth of a situation, but hear so many distortions of that truth that it makes you sad about our human race. I have a personal example of a family member that you might find interesting. When I was a teenager, my mother told me that her father had killed a man in self-defense when he was seventeen years old. A fortyish year old man had tried to rob him and pulled him off his horse and cut him with a knife. My grandfather shot and killed him due to fear for his life. The sheriff came to my grandfather's home and told him that he knew this was in self-defense and the local people would easily understand because this man was well known for being a troublemaker and had been in trouble with the law often before. There was no arrest or even a trial. The sheriff did recommend that my grandfather leave town for a few months because the family of the man he killed also had a reputation for retaliation. My grandfather went out west and worked on a cattle ranch for over three months and then returned home. He returned home with the passion to become a minister so he could help others for the rest of his life and to hopefully indicate his willingness to help others. He was successful for over forty years and was well respected for his ability. He was very well read and a pleasure to talk to.

A few years after my mother told me about my grandfather killing this robber in self-defense, I happened to be working in the area of where my grandfather grew up and started his career of ministry. There was an older man there, and we began talking. I mentioned that my family had some roots in this rural area. He asked me what their names were, and when I mentioned my grandfather, he remarked, "Oh yeah, he murdered a man here in the early 1900s!" He said nothing about the fact that there was no arrest, no trial, and the crime was deemed self-defense, or the forty years that my grandfather had been a minister and had never been in any trouble! I was appalled that this was what this man had been thinking about and, I am certain, talking about for all this time. It is just another example how we focus on anything negative about others so we will look good by comparison. The idea behind this type of thinking is to reduce everyone to the level of their mistakes so that our own don't seem so bad.

It is now time to move to our next to last but even more difficult level of forgiveness than we have experienced thus far. It is now time to deal with forgiveness needed due to family!

There is a well-known saying: "No one can hurt you like family"—as if this is such a great revelation! The only reason that family can seem to hurt you more is because they know you better than anyone. We spend years with our family in very close quarters much of the time, so there are few secrets among family members, especially in the early years while still living at home. So they have the most "ammunition" to unload on you if they choose to do so. You also have a great deal of knowledge of their shortcomings, so it could escalate to a war, but then everyone loses. A great stress reducer is to have positive relationships with your family, and a great stress increaser is when you have negative relationships with family. Not only can family hurt you but so can anyone who knows you.

People who don't know you can't hurt you because they don't know you! There are billions of people who cannot hurt me emotionally because they don't know or care to know me. So why worry about them? They might do me physical harm, but they can't do the emotional harm that someone can who really knows you.

Now that we have established that hardly anyone can need forgiveness more than our family, we need to determine how best to do that. As before, for your sake, just forgive them! I have always been amazed how families can be close for years and then fall apart over Grandmother's bed or Grandfather's old pistol! Probably neither item is worth much, but it can cause a rift in wonderful families. Inheritance time is another big cause of family stress. I personally believe that it is not good to allow your children to think they are going to inherit anything from you of any material value. That way they might not "pull the plug" to your life-giving machine in the old folks home if you have given them the right to do so. I have told my children for all of their life that I did not intend to leave them anything of much value other than a few personal items, and often personal items are really not worth much money—only the memories that might be associated with that item. An exception to this might be if you have a child or grandchildren or other relatives who might have a special need that could be benefited by your estate. My children and now my granddaughter always ask if they can have my room if I croak. I actually plan to live to be 120 years old if my health holds, so they are going to have to wait for a few years yet. There is a 200th reunion of the Oregon Trail horseback ride coming up in 2043 that I plan to attend and hopefully ride either my horse or a buggy the entire way. My daughters quickly told me how old I would be at that time, so I said, "Well, your husbands will probably be dead by then, so you can come along and take care of me!"

I have taught my children about God, given them as good a home as I was capable, and saw that they were able to get at least a college education, so I just don't feel this overwhelming obligation to leave them anything that might not be good for them...like money. So when I die, if they are still alive, they will not be fighting over anything of any value, especially after they see that my "room" is not such a treasure. I even have my funeral planned. I plan to donate my body, maybe to the "Body Farm" here in Knoxville or to Vanderbilt like my mother did. The funeral cannot last more than twenty minutes and will spend most of that time talking about my family, at least one song that I have sung to my children for years to put them to sleep, "Jesus Loves Me," fresh-baked chocolate-chip cookies with ice cream, and lots of laughter. I have even told my children to come over to my casket and say, "You know, you really were *despicable!*" and watch to see if the corners of their mouths turn up in a smile. I have even composed the poem that I want my granddaughter to say (she already has it memorized, and I am not certain that is a good thing). I composed this masterpiece after assisting in the speaking at the funeral service of one of my favorite uncles. My part was the "comedy" of his life, and he had plenty of stories that made us laugh. I did the same for my grandmother, and we still laugh about some of the unique things about her. (She was a midwife for over thirty years in the hills of Tennessee, where there was only one doctor in the entire county. She was trained by her mother, who also served as a midwife for an additional thirty years.) I know you are just dying to know about the poem that is to be read at my "celebration of life." I hope your eyes don't fill up so much with tears that you can't read, because we need to get back to forgiveness. Here goes: "Violets are blue, roses are red, you look dreadful, because you are dead!" That will really make me happy, especially if all two to four people who attend my funeral laugh. I have set aside enough money if we have to hire pall bearers in case all my friends are dead or too old to carry me without dropping me or if they are still willing to even let people know that they knew me. Actually when you donate your body, they take the body right away, so I might only have an empty casket buried. I also decided to order a cheap pine casket online and keep it in my attic so it would be ready. If you order almost anything online it most often will come with a great deal of assembly required, so maybe some of my relatives can be persuaded to assemble the casket to give them something to do prior to the funeral.

    Back to forgiveness—for the most difficult part of all, which may be considered by some as impossible: Forgive even your enemies!

OUR STRESS IS KILLING US: MONEY-BACK GUARANTEED SOLUTIONS

You may think that since I have told you I have had a blessed life, I don't even know what it is to have an enemy and certainly not more than one. I am sad to say that there is more than one, and sometimes they can be from your own family. Now these enemies may not be willing to come to my home to terminate me, but if someone did plan to do that and needed directions, they would not only tell them the way, but lead them here. I have even had to prepare a letter to give to others so that if I die under suspicious circumstances, they are to consider this enemy first. I have been advised by people who were somewhat knowledgeable about the situation with this enemy to "watch my back" and make certain to protect myself from physical harm. I have had one enemy accuse me of a crime that would have sent me to prison for fifteen years and would have totally ruined my life. I was able to stop that lie quickly by taking a police-administered lie detector test, so the accusation stopped at the interview stage and never made it to the investigation stage, which would have been followed by the grand jury stage, and then a trial if I had not done so well on the lie detector test. My lawyer advised me not to take the police-administered one, but I was leaving on a two-week trip to Australia (to horseback ride in the Snowy River mountain area), and I did not want that "anvil" hanging over my head. Fortunately, that accusation, which could have been so devastating, was averted. I even went back the next day to file false accusation charges, and the police said they would take my report, but they had too many other "real" crimes to ever get to my case. Luckily nothing ever came of any of this except the incredible stress I was under. My own lawyer asked me why she didn't have to come bail me out of jail because I had attempted some sort of physical retaliation on this person, and I replied that I had nothing to gain from doing anything physical but practically everything to lose.

One day I was visiting two different customers in two different small cities here in East Tennessee. I had known these customers for several years. We often went to lunch together or just talked privately about our families. I was relating some of my troubles, and I almost fell onto the floor when the first one asked me, "Do you want me to kill them for you?" Then he said he would make it look an accident and would do it for only $500 in cash! I knew this guy was a little "rough around the edges," but he had an important position in this small town, and I never dreamed that these words would come from him. Of course, I laughed it off as a joke and never went to lunch with him again. A few years later I was working in the emergency room of the new hospital in that small town, and I asked about him. I was told that he had been found dead due to some suspected criminal activity. Later that same day of the first offer of "Murder for Hire," I was visiting the second business, and the lady there and I were discussing my trouble well after she had told me all of hers. She also asked if I wanted this person killed. I was beginning to wonder if I was in a bad dream, and I hoped to awaken from it! She related that her husband knew people who would terminate this person for $500 cash! I thought life must certainly be cheap in this part of the world. I would never have suspected that either of these people would have even joked about something so serious. If that could have happened to me, then it must really be easy to find someone to cause someone else harm if you are looking for them. It is not too unusual for the police to set up "stings" on this type of crime, and it is always amazing who the person is that is doing the hiring.

Unfortunately, I have others who would qualify in the enemy category. Here I am having gone from thinking that everyone in my life liked me when I was a teenager to having people who might not harm me themselves but would be pleased if something did happen to me. So, I do have some idea of what it is like to have enemies.

I have had many patients tell me such horrific accounts of their abuse that it is really asking almost more than a person can even be capable of to ask them to forgive the abuser. The abuser does not deserve forgiveness, unless they ask for it, and I would recommend that you not hold your breath until they do. I would also ask you to realize that they will never, ever ask for forgiveness, so you might as well forgive them for yourself. Then you can graciously tell them that they are forgiven already if and when they come to ask forgiveness for their sake. Some of the stories were so horrible, but often the patient had the physical scars to indicate abuse. The more damaging and not readily observed emotional scars were even greater, by far, than the physical scars. One of my sweetest female patients, who exuded love and compassion, had been "sold" as a wife when she was twelve to a much older man because her mother needed the money. She became pregnant and had her first child by the time she was thirteen and did not even have a period prior to the pregnancy. This man abused her, but finally he died (hallelujah), and she remarried someone who was good to her. She was able to forgive without being able to hear an apology. Another patient was a grandmother by the time she was thirty. I saw her when she was thirty-three years old. She was a very attractive woman, and her daughter was also attractive and very mature-looking for her age. She should have had some maturity because she had a three-year-old and she was only sixteen, so she did not have the opportunity to have a normal teenage life. It appeared that she was not interested in taking care of her son, and her mother reinforced my observation. There had been sexual abuse in both generations.

I had a patient who had been referred to me by another patient, who came with her because she was so afraid of men. It took some time to calm her nerves, and the first few visits were difficult for her. She had been raped at age fourteen and was now raising the child who would not qualify to be called "love-child," but she loved him anyway. She was also very attractive (which seems to be a curse in some of our society) and was always in special education classes but loved to paint. She had not had any painting classes but was self-taught. On her next visit she brought in a painting that she had done for me! It was beautiful and now hangs in my office and is the item most often mentioned when others come to my office. Several have asked to purchase the painting or at least know who the artist is. Healthcare providers often receive small gifts that really mean a great deal when you realize that this person was thinking of pleasing you. None were ever considered a bribe because they had nothing to gain from such behavior, nor was this painting considered a "gift for a gift." She studied my office to see pictures of my black horse and mementos from my time on the Navajo Reservation (rez). She was from Phoenix and knew where I had studied in Monument Valley, Utah. She told me she might paint a picture of my horse for me and that she had some "risqué" ballerinas that she wanted to show me, but that she would keep them covered until I could see them.

On her next visit she did bring me a beautiful painting of my horse with an excellent representation of the southwest terrain in the background, as well as some Native American symbols all on the same canvas, done so very well. I could not believe that she took that amount of time to paint a unique painting like that. It is in my office and is one of my treasures. She also brought in a twelve-inch board that was forty-eight inches long (four feet) with four ballerinas painted on it. She did not bring it to the office covered as she said she would, and she should have, because all four ballerinas were full, face-on, shaved nudes that were shaped like only an artist could do. I learned that what an artist considered risqué would be considered pornographic at least in this case. I was actually embarrassed because all of my staff and patients had seen the long board painting so they knew what was on it, plus it had caused quite a stir among some of the male patients. I felt like everyone was thinking that I was taking "extra time" with this patient. It was graphic enough that in retrospect I should have asked that a female staff member chaperone us. When she left the horse painting, she asked if I wanted the ballerinas also, but I told her that I would not feel comfortable displaying it and really should not even be looking at it. After she left, the staff was laughing so hard about what attention the board had received all throughout the office. I see her seldom now because she is doing better, but she also had been abused most of her life. How difficult would it be for her to forgive when she has the child to rear who could bring back the memories of the abuse several times each and every day? Is it too much to ask her to forgive? Only she will know the benefit whenever she does.

Often when someone is asked to forgive another, they reply "I can forgive them for some of the things they did to me, but I will never forgive them for a part or parts of the offense!" This attitude is just as bad as remembering the entire scenario because when you remember the one major part, the other parts just flow right along with it. You are best at forgiving when you forgive everything, totally. To recall part is to recall all. Again you are doing this for *you* and not for them. I am not asking that you make this person your best friend or even associate with them if that is best for you, but do work diligently on forgiving and forgetting as much as you can. I mentioned that there is a benefit if you remember some of your errors so you will be stronger and won't repeat them, but it does you no good to say you are forgiving someone else but you still keep remembering. It is a "thought management" exercise to forgive and then to keep your mind from remembering because the fresh remembrance will soon overcome even your diligent efforts at forgiving.

Now we need to address an even more difficult task than forgiving enemies, like I shared with you (at great trepidation), to those who served in the military. They may have had "real" enemies, and their very effort was to kill them; often they were willing to give up their life in that effort. The VA just released numbers that an average of twenty-two veterans a day take their own life (this includes those up to sixty years old). In 2012 more than one soldier a day took their life who was actively involved in our current wars. One of the saddest realizations of the military dangers is that over four times as many soldiers killed themselves as soldiers who died in the bloody Vietnam War. Approximately 58,000 died in the active war, and over one-quarter million (250,000) of our soldiers took their lives mostly due to the trauma of the Vietnam War. That does not include those of even greater number who have had their entire lives damaged due to what they have seen. How can anyone ask a soldier to forgive the enemy when they were trained to hate and kill them? What a huge task that is! My heart truly grieves when I think of their pain, as it does when I reflect on anyone who is in such a place in their life where the only good option is to get out of this life by suicide. Is there anyone on this earth who can truly understand how much pain they are in? Once they have actually committed suicide, their pain is over, but their family suffers forever. I have some dear friends whose parents committed suicide, and they talk freely of their concerns that they might be prone to do the same thing.

I considered suicide for a very short time in my life due to my migraines. The pain was so great over one or the other of my eyes, I could easily have put a bullet or an ice pick or a knife there because the pain of doing so could not possibly be worse than the current pain. When you are lying there with so much pain due to the pounding of the blood flowing through the vessels and you can hear and feel each and every heartbeat in your head just immediately behind your eyes, then you are praying as you have never prayed before that nothing "pops" in your brain. You know that this hemorrhage will allow blood to flow out into the brain tissue right in the front where much of your cognitive thinking is done. Blood, when out of its containing vessels, is "poison" to the brain tissue and can turn you into a vegetable. I, like many, would rather be dead than to be unable to take care of myself. I often tell my patients that some of their illness, if uncontrolled, will give them a life where they plan their week around all the doctor's appointments, and to some that is worse than death.

I implore you military personnel who may be suffering so greatly with PTSD that you strongly consider beginning to forgive the officers who have had a negative impact on your career—they also are human and often scared to death that they might make the wrong decision that could cost you your life. What I do is nothing and not worthy to be compared to what an officer has to do in "harm's way." I seldom even see a patient who is in a position where my limited ability could cause them to die, but military staff faces it every day. I cannot project my active imagination far enough to be where they are or where you are now.

The next step is to forgive your peers, which is another stretch because the actions of your peers in the military could cost you your life also. True teamwork is evident in military situations and is far more important than teamwork on the "outside." Non-military teams that don't work together well may miss a deadline, lose the race, or fail in their goals, but the results are very seldom deadly to others as it is in the military.

Then comes the difficult task of forgiving your family and friends who you may feel have let you down in your most stressful time. So very often we have no idea of what you are dealing with because you have to be there to know the stress level, and often because the person does not adequately share how bad and dangerous the situation is for fear of upsetting those at home. So the best thing is to just "clear the slate" with your family and friends and forgive them for everything they did to you and, probably even much greater, what they did *not* do for you. Most often they did not ask for your forgiveness and still don't understand, so it is best for you to forgive them. If others don't understand your situation, it is similar to asking a child to understand your pain unless you have a big bandage for them to see. That is why it is very therapeutic to put a Band-Aid on a child. One of my difficulties of suffering with migraines was that they did not require a bandage, or sling, or cast, so others could see that I had reason for indicating that I was in pain.

Now comes the most difficult part—how to forgive those who really did attempt to *kill* you. It goes back to forgiving yourself as well as others. You might have even contributed to an action where someone was killed who should not have been, by your action or inaction. You have to forgive yourself for that mistake before moving on.

A true enemy who is attempting to kill you, or at least damage you so much that you never make it back to fight again, is especially difficult to forgive. One thing that could help is to realize that they have been taught from childhood to hate Americans and to be prepared to give their life to take an enemy's life. This indoctrination can seldom be undone, and so this person will never give any quarter or ask for forgiveness. Again, I ask you to forgive yourself and anyone else in your life. There is really no other way to begin to heal this tragedy you have suffered. It will be difficult, but you are trained to overcome difficult situations, so please search among your skills to assist you in a life-saving project. Even if someone does not take their life, it can be ruined by not forgiving. If you cannot forgive, it will damage *any* personal relationship you may have, and a good, positive personal relationship will do wonders for you!

Please remember that I am asking you to forgive for selfish reasons! Do it for yourself! Many will NEVER apologize because of their nature—never apologizing for anything and always blaming someone else for anything that has ever gone wrong in their life. Others will not apologize because they honestly don't realize that they even need to do so. Often, when others do apologize, we attempt to quantify their "I'm sorry" quotient to see if they are truly regretful. We are too often desirous of the other person's suffering so we can see their pain is as much as we hurt from whatever they did that needs forgiving.

Sometimes we are wrong about another person hurting us. It is often a matter of perception. I know I have hurt others in my life without intending to. I remember when my girls were smaller (they were five years apart) and I would ask the older daughter to read a sign or do some math for me as we drove, and then I would ask the younger daughter to sing for us. Later, my older daughter told me that she thought I did not think she could sing well. I was devastated that I had hurt her feelings! I asked her why she had that impression, and she said that I always asked my younger daughter to sing but not her. I explained that due to the age difference, my younger daughter could not read yet or do any math, so really the only way she could "perform" was to sing. So going forward I made certain to include both in the singing.

One time I was having a party at my house. I remarked on how slender one of the men was and that I felt maybe we needed to see that he ate more, primarily as a way of letting him know how we all appreciated his effort to remain a weight that suited him. After the party I received a call from another party attendee. I had hurt her feelings because I made her feel badly about her extra weight when I mentioned the man's success. I apologized for making her feel badly, when really I did not feel I had done anything incorrectly. But it was more important to me for her to feel good about herself than it was for me to "push back" about what I really should not have had to apologize for.

Sometimes a good way to give forgiveness is to ask the other person to forgive you if you have not done something that could be perceived as warranting an apology. This is a "disarming" gesture because it lets the other person know that you value the relationship you have (or did have) and want it restored. It is even acceptable to ask forgiveness in the business world. I have done this numerous times. When you work as many years as I have around so many different people, you are going to offend someone at some time, especially if you are driven to succeed, so you are focused on your goals too much sometimes and not fully aware that others may not be.

When you do ask forgiveness, then please ask for total forgiveness. I have done this so much that I have it down pat. "I want to ask you to forgive me for everything I have ever done to you or failed to do for you. I'm sorry." That statement just about covers everything most of the time. After you have made that statement in a sincere manner, then "protect" yourself by that statement also. If they want to discuss whatever it was, they usually mean they want to relive the incident(s), and usually their memory of the situation is much greater than yours or what might have actually happened. Stick to your statement and just state that you are not going to rehash the problem but that you are sorry for everything.

I had an incident where some young men asked me to be a business consultant for their new business in exchange for 5% of the company. These were very outstanding young men whom I had known for some time. They were just beginning this computer consulting business and wanted to rent an office in one of the upscale business areas in town. I told them not to do it, to conduct business out of their home office until the revenue was sufficient to afford the monthly rent and expenses. Well, they did it anyway and then asked me to meet with them in their new office. When I went there for the meeting, they wanted me to sign a note for them to borrow money as a start-up capital fund. I refused to do it for two reasons. One, they did not take my advice and made a poor decision on renting upscale office space before they could afford it. Secondly, I knew that if the note could not be paid, I would be responsible for the total amount. None of these young men had very much income at all at this time, so the lender would come after me for the total amount. The leader of the group was very angry with me for no good reason. I wanted this business to succeed for them as well as for me, so I apologized to the leader for anything I did or did not do. His statement was he could not forgive me now, but he wanted to schedule a meeting so we could discuss it later. I told him that there would not be a "later"—this was it, and I was not going to apologize again or discuss the matter further. He later borrowed the money from his grandfather and bought everyone else out and worked the business by himself, which is what he should have done in the first place because he wanted to control everything anyway. I even hired him to do some computer work for DuPont in some hospital laboratories later.

The point I want to make is to either give forgiveness or ask forgiveness basically one time and then be done with it, even if the other party wants to prolong the matter. Sometimes we want to twist that proverbial knife in those who have offended us, even when they apologize, so we need to recognize that others may want to do the same. Don't do it. Cut it off right at the pass, because further discussion just opens those old wounds for knife twisting. Sometimes we state, "Well, I can forgive you for this but not for that." This is a 100% or nothing situation. If anyone chooses to hold on to one part, they will remember the whole, and you are right back where you started. The sooner the better when you are forgiving or asking forgiveness, which is a wonderful philosophy because the negative situation seldom ever gets better with time, but most often grows and grows until it is a major happening and could become unforgivable. I did a great deal of entertaining in my business career, and I had a boss tell me one time that if I was entertaining where wine or drinks were being provided, to always buy the first round because the party never gets any smaller! Same with forgiveness. "Go first."

The stress relief is wonderful when you selfishly forgive others! Now you don't have to worry about that, and you can even begin to appreciate that person more for who they really are. You must have known them some for them to hurt you, so the relationship could be a good one for you. At the very least, evaluate the decision of the wisdom of walking away from a gratifying relationship. When you remember any of the early situations that were unpleasant, just use "thought management" and think of the positives that may have come from that and put it behind you...forever.

I have learned the self-preservation of forgiveness, and it was not an easy lesson! There will be some individuals who will never forgive you no matter what you do to show your willingness to achieve it. I have apologized to some, and they have said, "I don't believe you" and I have asked, "What do you want me to do, cut myself and bleed?" With some of the people in my life, that was probably not a good question—the cutting and bleeding could have been terminal! But some people are not going to forgive...ever. What I learned that has served me so very well is to get to the point in my life *that I no longer care what this person thinks of me.* I evaluate my life by what *most* others think of me, and if that is positive, then the person not willing to give me an even break because of what happened in the past becomes someone that I define as not important enough to me to worry about what they think of me. This is such a catharsis when you reach that level of not allowing what they think of you to concern you one little bit. Often others overestimate their importance to you or others in their life. We are all important to this world, but we are not important to every person, even if we have known them for many years. Actually, the person can still be very, very important to you, but their *opinion* of you is not.

A temptation with this stress-freeing attitude is that we might be so good at this attitude that we do something to make them think less of us. Please resist that because you are just attempting to protect yourself here, so stay with the "selfish" program of looking out for you and making your life more livable. If you do attempt to make things worse, it puts you in a negative situation and mind-set, which is contrary to good emotional health.

Now that you have successfully achieved a threshold where you no longer are concerned about what this person thinks of you, it is possible to go to an even better place of stress relief! You can't hurry this process; you must successfully achieve the first level, where it matters not to you what that person thinks of you. The second step is even more important! This is really a great "leap" to help you. You get to the point that you don't care what they think about **anything**! Their opinion about other relationships, the weather, politics, money, the future, or anything on this earth is of no interest to you. They have proven that they are not willing to work on the most important relationship issues, so it is "mind freeing" when this person's opinion becomes a non-issue. You have done the best you can, so you now move on to finding other positive relationships in your life. If you are successful in achieving this level of still caring for the person but not their thoughts on anything, then I know you will feel some relief. This self preservation process is the technique that the very intelligent young lady who had such a serious skin condition used to overcome much of her stress that was discussed earlier.

Bullying is unwanted, aggressive behavior among not only school aged children but also adults that involves a real or perceived power imbalance. Bullying includes actions such as making threats, spreading rumors, attacking someone physically or verbally, and excluding someone from a group on purpose. If **anyone** is bullying you at any time then report it immediately! It will only become worse! Fortunately, our world is more aware of the dangers of tolerating bullying, so report it. Then forgive them for _your_ sake.

Holiday Stressors

Holidays are some of the most stressful days of the year and are dreaded by many. Often the biggest stress is from our "marketing world" as discussed earlier about Valentine's Day. My stress level was greatly reduced when I told all adults that I was only going to buy Christmas gifts for the children. This does still cause me some stress because some of my family enjoy Christmas for months and do not agree with my stance on this, but it is not because they are expecting something from me. They just consider me out of touch with reality, or at least that is probably the best phrase they use for me. Most adults in the U.S. don't really *need* anything. One reason I enjoy small children is that they enjoy any gift even if it is not expensive. Many adults are disappointed if they don't get the keys to a new car in their stocking because it takes quite a gift to impress others now. I remember buying a very powerful electric generator one summer for my father's family because they have several ill people in their home. They said "I thought you didn't believe in Christmas!" I remarked that this was not Christmas, "but it is a gift for you."

One reason I enjoy Thanksgiving so very much is that there is no gift-giving pressure unless you count the obligation to bring food. I do so enjoy the fellowship with family during that time of preparation and dining. The conversation is so heart-warming and is far better for us than the meal. I remember one year when my immediate family decided that we would just go out to a restaurant for a "nice Thanksgiving dinner." That did not work because we ate out often enough that this was just another meal. With our propensity for eating out in our society, now just having a home-cooked meal at the dining table is almost a rarity. I have been blessed with eating in some of the finest restaurants in the U.S. when I was working in the corporate world, but none of those meals was as good as a home-cooked meal. I absolutely love going to gatherings where the food is pot-luck! I have never found better food to eat anywhere or at any time that equals that type of spread—home-cooked by others who have a well-tested, favorite recipe, but even at such an excellent meal, it is the social interactions that are most important.

When I take home-cooked food to these pot-luck dinners, I take cornbread from a recipe from my father. He won many blue ribbons in his local county for his cornbread, biscuits, and other items. Everyone who eats his cornbread loves it, because it reminds them of their childhood. One time I was having a party and someone brought in some cornbread that rivaled my father's! I asked her the secret, and she said she just used a cornbread mix out of a box (which a "real" home cook would never do) and added a stick of butter to every making! I now do that and my father's recipe is even better! So my stress level is lowered when I am invited to a pot-luck because I take the same thing if I have time to cook. In reality, I often go without taking anything because those who do bring food always bring too much. I do attempt to clean up afterward to make up for my not cooking. I very, very seldom cook the cornbread for me because it is so good that I eat too much of it myself.

High Expectations

Sometimes our expectations of the holiday season are too high. We see so many movies and TV shows about families that are unrealistic, so we expect to achieve this level of happiness at every holiday. So it is best for your stress level to just focus on what good you can get out of the gathering because often the times are not that pleasant—no one knows you like family. And they too often remember negatives times and want everyone to know that they remember them. So many people are unhappy now that they want everyone else to be like them. Just don't play that game with them. It is amazing what ignoring someone can do for keeping the peace at a family gathering.

I recently went to a meeting where we were planning our high school reunion, and everyone was having a marvelous time. All of a sudden, out of the blue, one member said, "I remember running all over you in our football game in the eighth grade." He must have hit me especially hard because I don't remember anyone running over me the entire eighth grade. Then he remarked how well he remembered the game. The final score was seven to six, and with that score it is difficult to label that game as one side running all over the other. I do remember the game but not the score because it was not important to me. But it certainly was important to him. Often situations like that are brought up at family holidays. Actually, we should relish our family holidays because they are about the only time extended families get together anymore—Thanksgiving, Christmas, sometimes the 4th of July, planned reunions, weddings, and funerals.

Positive Attitude

"Attitude determines your altitude not your aptitude!" is from Zig Ziglar, so I didn't make that up. It is difficult to have a positive attitude today, but it is well worth the effort to become more positive. This outlook will make seemingly "bad" situations less unpleasant and can significantly reduce your stress level. There is much here to help with a positive attitude like a good night's sleep, feeling more energetic, and accomplishing tasks.

Love Runs Downhill

Another stress reducer is to realize fully that your children will never, ever love you as much as you love them! They may love you a great deal and learn to respect you also, but if you are expecting them to love you as much as you love them, it will set you up for stress-relief failure.

We parents are very important to our children, but our importance drops greatly as they mature, and if you are aware that this is a natural process, then it can reduce your stress. A parent's importance to their children really drops when they have their own children, and sometimes that is very difficult for us parents to handle, especially if we expect our children to love us as much as we love them. Now, one wonderful thing that happens often when your children have their own children is that their respect for you often increases, so that is some consolation. Please don't ever set yourself up for failure by asking your child to decide between you as a parent or their child, because the response (which is totally natural) is that you are not even on the radar screen if there has to be a choice.

My granddaughter and I are very close because I have assisted in rearing her and get to spend a good of time with her. So right now I am still an important male in her life, but my importance to her will diminish in certain natural stages so that I almost fall off of her list. Every other significant male in her life will push me down the list. First it will probably be a male teacher or coach. Then it will be a boyfriend. Then certainly I will drop precipitously when she marries. The final drop will be if she has a son. So I am already prepared for my "fall from grace" position, but I am relishing every moment of the time I do seem somewhat important to her.

Smile—Embodied Cognition (Fake It Till You Make It)

"Embodied cognition" is a term that I just read in some article to attempt to dress this work up with big words that actually mean, "Just smile until you feel like smiling!" How does that work? Well, normally when you smile, others smile back, and that brings on good feelings, which we all need as often as possible. I have so often found that a smile even diffuses a situation when I have made a mistake when driving. I was able to attend a three-day, very specialized telephone skills course during my career. One of the techniques to make you "smile" on the phone is to look at your face in a mirror as you are talking, because the person on the other end can actually tell if you are smiling by just your tone of voice and/or inflection.

A goal that has greatly reduced my stress and enhanced my life both professionally and personally is to smile more often and attempt to better the other person's day, if possible. The giving of yourself to others cannot be overemphasized because it really does reduce your stress to help someone else reduce their stress.

Overcoming Sorrow

We all either have sorrow right now or we will have it sometime in our lives. There is no escape from this situation, and it truly hurts when we have to deal with whatever sorrow we are going through. There is a technique that can help us deal with sorrow that is golden.

First we must understand that we can only feel sorrow for someone or something if we have known them closely or possessed the item we may have lost. When there is a tragedy in some other part of the world that the media tells us about over and over, we are sad but not to the level we would be if we actually knew that person. I don't know what it is like to lose a father, but I know what it is like to have a mother die. I don't know what it is like to lose a million-dollar item because I have never had anything of that value (and I doubt if I will because of all the stress that goes with such a purchase).

The point I am so poorly attempting to make is that you can only feel sorrow for something if you have had the joy of experiencing it! There is a very useful formula that helps me tremendously in these situations.

Sorrow = Joy

I hope that does not disappoint you in its simplicity, but this formula says that your sorrow can only equal the amount of joy by knowing that person you have lost to death or divorce or desertion. If there was no joy, then there is no sorrow. If it was a caustic relationship, there can actually be some joy of them being out of your life, and that is a humbling thought when you think anyone would be glad that you are not in their life.

Now if you will look back at this formula, which states that our sorrow can only equal what joy you had, then you can decide what part of the equation or which side of the equal sign you want to focus on. To greatly reduce your current sorrow and stress level, cause your mind to focus most of the time on the "joy" part. Where you put your emphasis will greatly facilitate your movement through the grieving process. I have had someone step out of my life who is very important to me, so I use this equation almost daily by remembering the good times and the joy that made me even have *any* sorrow that I no longer have that relationship. I told this person, "I have a wonderful life, and I would like for you to be a part of it, but if you choose not to be a part of my life, then I am still going to have a wonderful life." This simple system will help you more than you realize, when and if you start concentrating on the positive side of this "life" equation.

Increase Success

You Are Already Successful

Another source of stress is when we see the rich and famous and we think we are not successful and therefore less worthy than they are. It helps greatly to realize that you are already successful and that others envy what you now have. Even the poorest of those living in the U.S. are light-years ahead of much of the world. If you have a job, you are a success. If you have a family, you are a success. If you are a good parent, you are a success at the most important job you have. If you are in good health and/or have access to healthcare, you are a success. The list could go on and on because we use the inappropriate standard to measure ourselves by. If you are doing the best job of everything you can and are making the best decisions you can (even if you fail over and over), then you are a success.

Be a Decision Maker

If you can make decisions quickly, your stress level will go down also. That is one way of determining if a person is really overstressed, if they can't seem to make a decision. All of your life you have been making decisions, and most of them have been good ones. We tend to focus on our mistakes even if others do not. We often fail to realize that we humans all make mistakes, but we cannot dwell on the negative ones. If I were to list all the mistakes I have made over my life, it would be longer than this entire book. I have missed so many wonderful opportunities because I decided not to follow up on them.

The peace that comes from being a decision maker is that you can correct your course quickly. Keep in mind that making a decision to delay a decision—as long as you have a reasonable time frame—is still a wonderful practice. You can always make the decision to reverse or alter your first decision. If you have 80% of the facts needed to make a decision, go ahead and make the decision. If something comes to light from the 20%, you can always alter your course. Very seldom is there anything of importance in the 20% or you would have already considered it.

You can even play the odds in your favor if you are a decision maker. If you have a choice of three decisions, your odds of being correct is one-in-three or 33%. After you find that the first decision was not the correct or best one, then you can discard that one from your list, and now your odds have just improved to one-of-two or 50%. If that decision is not the best one, you are down to one-to-one or 100% chance of being correct, so the stress-lowering benefit of making a decision is tremendous.

It is best for you to realize that most of your decisions are correct and to have the confidence to know that, tell yourself that often, and keep getting better at making decisions. Always remember that nearly all of your decisions are correct, but you just want to keep improving. If you misplace your car keys, that does not mean you are a failure for that entire day. You decided to get up, drink a great deal of water, eat a good breakfast, take care of your morning chores at home and at work, you make a good decision at lunch to eat and relax for a few minutes...until you realize that losing your keys was really a small mistake. Then you can make a decision to keep your keys in a certain place so you can always find them there in case of an emergency.

Encourage Others

If you want to be more effective at reducing stress, then do something for others! You may be asking, "How can I do that when I am so beat up right now?" Share some of your story with others in a manner that brings them amusement. This will also be therapeutic for you. Someone somewhere is looking up to you, and that is a super scary thing to know. I remember the shock I experienced when a young mother told me that her young son looked up to me as if it were yesterday! I could not believe it. So just look around for someone who is in more trouble than you are and make their day by some word of encouragement. The joy this gives you (in addition to what it does for them) is immeasurable and greatly reduces your stress level.

We all need encouragement because this world will not do much in that department. Even if you win some type of award, the glory is short-lived, and often others are not glad you received it. Most of the world does not want to rejoice with you, but others want to hear your sad story so they can revel in your grief and troubles.

Write Notes

A handwritten note is almost equivalent to baking someone a cake and delivering it in person in today's society. Cards are so thoughtful, but you really read what the sender wrote in their own handwriting. Some card senders at least underline some of the sentiment written there. To go even further, do the entire card by hand, those of you who have any artistic talent (which I don't, so I have to just rely on the wording). Unfortunately, my penmanship is poor, but still I feel that others would rather struggle to read personal handwriting than a preprinted card. If you even think of doing some kindness for someone then please do it right then or else you may forget it. I have found that anytime I am having a "bad day" the best thing I can do is to do something for someone else.

Phone Calls

Make a quick phone call to cheer someone up even if you know they will not be able to answer. It will be so pleasant for them to pick up the message later. We all need our spirits lifted at times, and just a quick personal gesture will be more appreciated than we can imagine until someone does that for us. It is similar to not realizing how much it means to reach out to others when they are ill until we become ill and know how it brightens our entire day to hear from a good friend.

Give, Give, and Give

In the years 2010, 2011, and 2012, I was able to give approximately $2.5 million dollars in free services to the medically underserved of East Tennessee from my Healthy Life Clinics. That was the best $2.5 million *I never made*! Actually, I needed some of that money to keep my clinics viable, but much of it was a decision to "lose money" if it meant helping others. Our staff at Healthy Life Clinics knew coming in that we would be doing a good deal of work that we would never be reimbursed for. Actually, many medical facilities give much more than that away, but we were a small company with no more than twenty-five employees and only slightly more revenue than we gave away. This was not including the free tables in each clinic and other works that the staff performed. This was one of the greatest blessings of my life that I did for **me**! Yes, it did benefit others, many others, but most of all I love what it did for me!

In 2011, I was given two wonderful awards that I really did not deserve as a businessman, but I feel they came my way due to the type of work I attempted to do, especially at a time when our nation was severely struggling with our healthcare provider system for the medically underserved. I regret that I was not able to do more, and maybe someday I will. Please don't think I am bragging about what I did because it was my pleasure. The first award was "Outstanding Alumni for 2011" for Walden University, where I obtained my doctoral degree. At one of the smaller schools I attended, they have several outstanding alumni each year, so I assumed this much larger school (with over 61,000 alumni from 110 countries) would have many awards that year. When they flew me to their headquarters, I was given the VIP treatment and I thought this was costing Walden too much money for all of us. At the award banquet I found out that I was the only one who had been given that award for 2011. I was elated, overwhelmed, and humbled at the same time. I personally did not deserve this, and I am totally convinced that my decision to serve the medically underserved brought about this wonderful award. I believe that if I had been as successful in another type of endeavor, I would not have been selected. The award ceremony was so very wonderful, and so I decided to go to the graduation ceremony since I had chosen not to do that when I graduated fourteen years earlier.

I am so glad that I did, because former President Bill Clinton was the speaker, so then I was even more impressed with Walden for getting such a well-known person as a speaker for the graduation ceremony. What was most impressive about him was his relating that because of his foundation to help reduce AIDS in third world countries, they were able to reduce the cost of providing the appropriate drugs to the patients from $3.5 thousand per patient per year to now down to under $100.00 per patient per year by eliminating some of the graft from the system and using competitive bidding on the drugs. His work made my work seem like nothing in scope, but I have had such pleasure in helping others that I have very few regrets of the past few years.

Walden University also had a "Scholars for Change" contest that year where you submitted a short video telling your story, which would be on the Walden Website for others to view and vote for their favorite. I was extremely busy seeing patients and attempting to keep my other clinics staffed and operating sufficiently, and I did not have time to do this work even with the $5,000 award that would be split between my clinics and any donation I selected. Fortunately, I had two summer interns who attended where I worshiped who were super sharp young ladies. I called them in and gave them my appropriate passwords and gave them full responsibility to submit our work to this contest. They did it all, and the only time I spent on this important project was telling them about it and the few minutes when they set up a camera in my office to interview me. They also interviewed themselves, other employees, did all scripting, editing, and even added original music from one of my very best friends and the father of two of the five young people who finally became involved in the project.

When I went to the award banquet, they showed the video that these wonderful, talented young people had put together, after introducing me but before I was to give a short speech. During the introduction, it was announced that the video about our work with the medically underserved was in third, with some votes to still come in. At the end of the voting time, we were declared a winner! And it was because of the work we were all attempting to do for others. The five young people put their heart and soul into this project because they knew that they were able to assist us in giving to others. How many high school students are able to win $5,000 for charity? We gave $2,500 to Remote Area Medical Corps, based here in Knoxville. If you want to know about one of the best works for others in the entire United States as well as other parts of the world, just visit ramusa.org and spend a few minutes seeing what they do. That $2,500 donation from Walden University covered the expenses for hundreds of patients for dental, vision, and medical care. Stan Brock is the one who started Remote Area Medical (RAM), and he used to be the "muscle man" on Wild Kingdom. He is truly an amazing man. He does not take a salary and lives in an old schoolhouse that was built in the 1920s that RAM leases from Knoxville City schools for a dollar a year. These young people have touched so many lives by their efforts to assist in any way they can to help others.

The other award that my medical mission work gained for me

was the national award for Entrepreneur of the Year over fifty years old. This award was from a part of the U.S. Dept. of Labor's Small Business Association's SCORE division. SCORE is a group of successful business men and women who work as volunteers (for no money) helping others succeed in business. This is another wonderful group of people who use their skills to help others. Hundreds of small businesses were nominated for this national award. My mentor in this work was Charles Christiansen, a very successful businessman who consults all over the world helping others for free. He was eighty years old when we went to Washington, DC to accept this national award. Once again I thought that there would be several other winners in this same category and that the winner would be announced at the banquet, so I really was thinking of what excuses I could give for not winning the "big" award and how pleased I was to just be a part of such a wonderful celebration. This was even a black tie affair, so my thoughts were, "Great, now I have to either rent or purchase a tuxedo just to be a runner-up." Mr. Christiansen would never allow me to give him anything for all the many hours and effort he expended in helping me start my business. When I went to purchase a tuxedo, they were having a buy-one-get-one-free! I was able to convince him to take the other free one because I certainly did not need two such outfits. When we got to the banquet at the Ronald Reagan International Building, the security was tremendous. I felt we were in the safest place we could be while there in Washington, DC. As it turned out the medical mission work that Chuck and I started was the only one selected for this category! What an honor! Again, I know in my heart of hearts that I am not a better businessman than the hundreds of others who were nominated from across the nation, but I know it was the work that we were attempting to do for others. Chuck and I were the old guys, but we had a wonderful time. If you would like to know more, just go to the SCORE website for the Small Business Administration and type my last name into the search area to see the custom video they produced about the work Chuck helped me with. A year later Chuck was awarded some other wonderful award that would have been given to him by the President of the United States, but he chose not to go so he would have more time with his clients. I did everything to talk him into going and even volunteered to go with him as his "valet," but I was not successful. He has won so many awards for his efforts to help others already, and that is not why he does it. I failed to mention he has diabetes and has finally cut down to only forty-fifty hours a week instead of the sixty hours per week that he volunteered for years. There are twenty to thirty volunteers in the local SCORE chapter, but Chuck sees over 50% of all of clients in our county and several other counties as well as all across the U.S. and the world.

Summary

Stress Is Both Positive and Negative

The proper amount of stress is one of our best friends, but too much stress is one of our greatest enemies! If you recognize that we can't escape all stress on this side of the grave, then as long as you can channel, reduce, or eliminate the stress that comes our way on a daily basis, every day, then we honestly can have a much more fulfilled life. And even if we don't actually live longer we can know that our lives are better, as well as those around us, if we are able to control the level of stress in our lives.

Increase Energy

If we follow the normal, natural, healthy, money-saving suggestions about treating our bodies with the utmost respect for their wonderful capabilities and "partner" with our body, we will find that the world is a better place. I greatly encourage you to try all the suggestions to the very best of your ability for a full thirty days, and then evaluate where you were a month ago compared to where you are after the "30 day change of habits trial."

Positive Attitude Toward Life

A positive attitude toward life and what is happening to you is tantamount to your success and contentment in this world. Even the negative times can and most often do have a positive component, but we might just have to dig a little deeper to find it. The rewards of a positive attitude are so great, you will regret the time you have **not** had this wonderful attitude.

Reach Out

Please make every effort to be good to others. The world needs you to do that. Your family needs for you to do that. You need to do that because the rewards you will receive are so lovely in the betterment of your relationships that you will automatically look for ways to do more. Even a smile is worth so very much to others. Those contacts with others, by any means available, that have a positive effect on the recipient are always less than the good feeling that *you* have by taking the time from your stressful life to be good to others.

Be Good to Yourself

Don't ever forget to be good to yourself in the process of reducing your stress level. YOU are very important to this universe, and everything you do has some impact somewhere on someone, so please make it as positive an impact as you can. This is another place where you will never regret taking care of your own needs, as well as when you are seeing to the needs of others. Remember, forgiving others is always good for **you!**

Use Stress to GROW!

Stress is one of our greatest blessings because it causes us to do our very best, so look at it as an ally that is here to help you. As soon as you recognize that your ally is becoming your enemy, then make certain you are following the simple principles listed here, plus your own set of principles that improve on what is here. You can, you know, because **YOU** are someone extra special, and the day you were born was a wonderful day!

www.ingramcontent.com/pod-product-compliance
Lightning Source LLC
Chambersburg PA
CBHW071147160426
43196CB00011B/2030